GW00359934

Michael Glasspool studied medicine at Cambridge University and the Middlesex Hospital, London. After a period spent in general surgery he trained as an ophthalmologist at Moorfields Eye Hospital. He then became Senior Registrar to the Eye Department at Westminster Hospital until his appointment as Consultant Ophthalmic Surgeon at Orpington Hospital. He has written many articles and papers and two specialist books on the eye, *Problems in Ophthalmology*, and *Atlas of Ophthalmology*. He has lectured in Sri Lanka and been interviewed on British television and radio and in the press. His hobbies are classical guitar and painting.

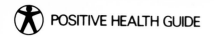
POSITIVE HEALTH GUIDE

EYES
Their problems
and treatments

Michael Glasspool, FRCS, DO

MARTIN DUNITZ

© Michael Glasspool 1984
First published in the United Kingdom in 1984 by Martin Dunitz
Limited, London

British Library Cataloguing in Publication Data

Glasspool, Michael
    Eyes: (Positive health guide)
    1. Eye
    I. Title   II. Series
    612'.84   QP475

ISBN 0-906348-55-2
ISBN 0-906348-54-4 Pbk

Phototypeset in Garamond by Input Typesetting Ltd, London
Printed by Toppan Printing Company (S) Pte Ltd, Singapore

CONTENTS

INTRODUCTION

So many of my patients ask me detailed questions about their eyes and treatments that I have been aware for a long time of the need for a book answering all those queries and doubts. I have written this book as a guide to the normal eye and the changes that most often happen with ageing and disease. It is not a do-it-yourself manual but it does answer the questions that are likely to occur to you about your eyes, whether or not they need treatment at the moment. It should also help clarify any points made by your doctor or eye specialist if you have recently had an appointment and found it difficult to remember or take in everything you were told.

You will find in the first chapters that I give a fairly detailed description of the normal eye, its workings and the ways it should be treated. One point I should emphasize, which is a firm belief of mine and many other eye specialists: the term 'eye care' is all too easily abused. Most doctors believe that your eyes are quite capable of looking after themselves and do not need cosseting, as some people think. Of course they should be treated well, just as you buy the right sized shoes, clean your teeth or wash your hair. The advice I give in Chapter 4 will show that there is no need to take extra measures to 'preserve' your eyes.

Since everyone eventually needs glasses, at least for reading, I explain how these will help focusing problems and give advice on choosing between the different types of glasses and contact lenses. Your children's sight will certainly be of concern to you, and so I have dealt separately with the special problems occurring most often in children. These are naturally fewer than the disorders we tend to develop as we reach middle age and beyond. The book moves broadly from the common problems of youth and young adulthood to those of the middle years and old age. To help you find your way around I have given a short summary in Chapter 2 of the symptoms you may experience if you have any of these diseases. You will then be able to turn directly to the chapter which deals more fully with your symptoms.

Most people are familiar with the difficulties of living with failing sight; if our own eyesight does not deteriorate in later years, then we probably all know people who are partially sighted or blind. In the last chapter I give some practical advice on how to cope with the day to day problems and I point to the many organizations and facilities available for aid and support.

This is not a specialist book but a guide for everyone to the many troubles that can affect the eye. I hope I have given sufficient information to allay doubts you may have and to help you help your specialist make your treatment the most effective.

1 HOW YOUR EYES WORK

Many people reading this book will be doing so because either they or a relative or friend may be suffering from a particular eye problem. If you are in this group you will find it easier to follow if you have a basic understanding of your eyes and how they work – and this is what I hope this chapter will provide. Once you have grasped the mechanism, the anatomy of the eye is quite simple to remember.

How does the eye work?

The usual and most understandable way of describing the working of your eye is to compare it to a camera. At the front of the eye is the lens, held in place by surrounding muscle, which focuses on what you want to see. The exposure to light is regulated by the coloured iris expanding and contracting to allow the correct amount of light into the eye. All round the inside of the back of the eye is the retina, which acts like the light-sensitive film in the camera.

When the eye is relaxed and looking into the far distance the rays of light are focused on to the retina. If you wish to look at something nearer, perhaps at 6 ft (2 m), the focus of the lens is adjusted by the surrounding muscle, called the ciliary muscle. This process of focusing is called accommodation.

The retina, which is a mere 1/50 in (0.4 mm) thick, both changes light into electrical energy (rather as a light meter does) and processes this into coded impulses to be transmitted to the brain.

So, an image passing through the lens is transmitted from the retina to your brain. The impulses sent to the brain from the retina travel via the optic nerves, which pass from the front to the back of the brain before reaching the area that is responsible for vision. There is a complex mixing of the impulses so that the right side of your brain sees everything on your left, while the left side of your brain sees everything on your right. As in a camera, the image appears upside down on the retina, but your brain instantly converts it so that you see everything the right way up.

Your eyes move together and send the brain almost identical images. Your brain then joins these two images into a single mental picture. The slight difference in the images is needed to produce stereoscopic (three dimensional) vision. You can test this yourself by looking with one eye and then the other at a rectangular shape, for example, a matchbox, when you will notice the different views you get with each eye.

The anatomy of the eye

Each of your eyes is spherical and about 1 in (2.5 cm) in diameter. To get an idea of the whole anatomy, I shall describe the parts you can see first, and then the inside of the eye.

If you look in a mirror you will see that your eyelids cover about two-thirds of each eyeball (see the diagram opposite). Where the eyelids join beside the nose there is a small pink fleshy swelling and beside this is a thin fold of skin which is a remnant of the third eyelid that is found in some animals, but has no function in man.

The cornea is like a clear watch-glass which covers the central part of the eyeball. Through it you can see the coloured iris, in the middle of which is a hole, the black pupil. The colour of the iris varies from one person to another and depends on the amount of pigment that it contains. The darker your skin the browner the iris tends to be. Fair-skinned people often have so little pigment that the iris appears blue. The iris reacts to light by enlarging the pupil in dim light or by diminishing it in bright light.

The lens of the eye is suspended immediately behind the iris and is attached to a ring-shaped muscle, the ciliary muscle, which performs the act of focusing (see page 9). This is done by the muscle contracting to alter the shape of the lens, making it more spherical.

This process of accommodation is easily done when you are young. After the age of forty the muscle becomes weaker and the lens hardens, making accommodation more difficult, so that glasses are needed for close work. I describe this in more detail in Chapter 5.

The sclera or white of the eye surrounds the cornea and is covered by a thin, transparent membrane, the conjunctiva, which also lines the inside of the eyelids.

Inside the eye

Behind what you can see of the eye is the major part (see the diagram opposite), which consists of three layers:

1. The sclera or white of the eye forms the outermost coat, which is tough and protects the delicate linings inside.

2. The choroid is the middle layer. This is made up of blood vessels supplying the nutrition to the innermost layer.

3. The retina is a thin membrane which contains the cells that are sensitive to light and enable you to see. There are two types of retinal cells – cones and rods, so-called because of their shape.

    The cones, which allow you to distinguish colours, are distributed at the back of the eye and can only react to colours in daylight. They are concentrated especially in the area called the macula which is used for direct vision such as reading.

The outside of the eye

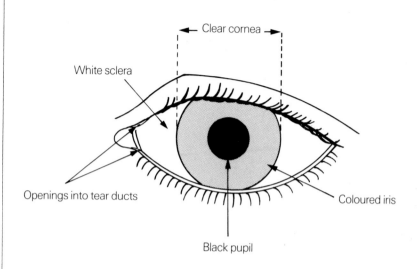

← Clear cornea →

White sclera

Openings into tear ducts

Coloured iris

Black pupil

The inside of the eye

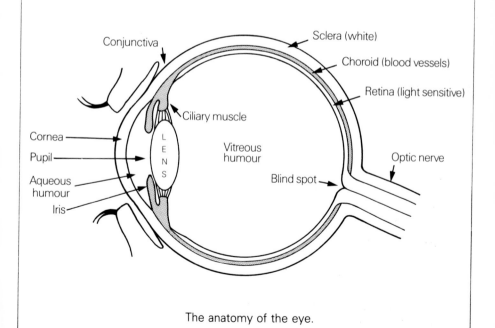

Conjunctiva

Sclera (white)

Choroid (blood vessels)

Retina (light sensitive)

Ciliary muscle

Cornea

Pupil

LENS

Vitreous humour

Optic nerve

Aqueous humour

Blind spot

Iris

The anatomy of the eye.

The rods, which are placed around the edge of the retina, come into use in dim light. Colour cannot be detected by rods, which explains why a scene lit only by moonlight appears colourless. The concentration of rods away from the macula is also the reason that you are able to see an object more easily in dim light when you look to one side rather than looking directly at it.

The movements of your eyes are controlled by the muscles attached to your skull. The optic nerves that transmit the impulses from the retina to the brain are a collection of separate nerve fibres rather like a telephone cable. However, whereas a telephone cable may contain several thousand wires, each optic nerve contains up to one million nerve fibres and yet is only 1/10 in (3 mm) across. Because of the complicated route of the optic nerves from the front to the back of the eye, it is often possible for a doctor to localize the site of illnesses within your brain by testing your vision.

The importance of tears

Tears are not produced when you cry; they are present in your eyes all the time and are essential for you to be able to see. Without them your eyes would become gritty and painful.

Tears, which are salty in taste, are produced by the tear gland in the upper lid. With each blink a film of tears is swept across the eye to keep it moist and remove dust. Tears also have some mild antiseptic properties which help to keep the eye clean. There is a steady supply of tears which may be increased by emotion when you cry or by getting something in your eye which makes it water.

The tear fluid drains constantly into the tear ducts, which are on the edges of the eyelids at their inner ends, and then through small channels into the nose. This explains why your nose runs when you cry and why you taste salt in your mouth as the tears run down on to the back of your tongue.

Behind the clear window of the cornea and in front of the lens lies a space which is filled with watery fluid called the aqueous humour, or fluid. This is quite different from the tears and supplies the nutrition to the lens and it maintains the shape of the eyeball by regulating the pressure inside it, like air in a balloon.

This brief description of the working and anatomy of the eye should make for easier understanding of both the simple disorders and the more severe and unusual diseases that I describe in this book. In the next chapter I describe the various symptoms that will help you identify which particular problem you may have; though as you will see, this is never an easy task.

2 SYMPTOMS OF EYE TROUBLE

Many different diseases that affect your eyes can produce similar symptoms, making it very difficult to decide what is your particular problem. This chapter is designed to help you find your way around this book by describing briefly what you will experience at first, what your problem may be, and how it will affect your eyes. The chapters dealing with each of the diseases explain the causes and treatments in more detail.

The first symptoms

All eye ailments begin with one or more of the following symptoms:

1. Sight disturbance
2. Discomfort or pain
3. Discharge from your eyes
4. Altered appearance of your eyes.

Sight disturbance

This is the most important symptom of eye disease, and is often the earliest and only indication that something is wrong. In order to separate the different causes you must decide how your sight has altered. By covering one eye at a time, compare the sight in both eyes. You will notice if the trouble affects one eye or both. Then check to see which of the following is closest to your own problem:

- Loss of vision
- Generalized blurring
- Central loss
- Peripheral loss
- Patchy loss
- Half vision
- Double vision
- Flashing lights and spots.

Loss of vision   Usually loss of vision is gradual as part of the eye ceases to work. Sudden loss is due either to an accident or to an interruption of the blood supply to the retina or brain. People with a longstanding gradual loss are apt to think they have sudden loss of vision when the good eye is suddenly closed – when a piece of grit gets in, for example. Although the loss of vision in the weak eye may have been slow it is noticed only now.

Generalized blurring A general blurring of all that you look at may indicate that you need glasses. This may be for distance viewing if you are short-sighted or for reading if you are over forty-five; or for both if you have astigmatism (Chapter 5).

Any stickiness or discharge from your eyes may blur your vision because of the abnormal tear film – like looking through a dirty window. This blurring will come and go as you blink and can be a sign of conjunctivitis (Chapter 6).

This type of loss of vision may occur with any inflammation within the eye such as iritis (Chapter 6).

An overall dimming of vision that comes on gradually is most frequently caused by cataracts (Chapter 9). Both distance and near vision are affected, although one may be worse than the other.

Central loss Loss of your central vision means you have a central blur or gap whenever you look directly at something. So words you are trying to read are absent although you are aware of the edges of the page, or a person's nose may seem to be missing, even though you can still see his or her ears. This is usually due to a change in the central part of the light-sensitive retina (Chapter 9).

Occasionally, in the early stage of central loss, you may notice slight kinks in straight lines, or letters on a page may appear slightly smaller.

Peripheral loss It is easy to overlook loss of peripheral or side vision because your central vision remains normal, so allowing you to read, sew, see a signpost or follow a golf ball. When loss of peripheral vision is gradual your brain learns to adapt to the blinkered view of life. This occurs with glaucoma (Chapter 8). You may first notice your loss of peripheral vision as you become clumsy, bumping into furniture or people in the street.

Sudden loss of side vision is usually obvious. It seems as if a curtain has been drawn over part of your vision. This is typical of retinal detachment (Chapter 10).

Patchy loss This is difficult to detect if it happens in only one eye. The sight in the normal eye compensates for the defective areas in the poor eye. Only when both eyes are affected can you notice the change in your sight. You can test for this loss by looking steadily at a cross drawn in the centre of a piece of graph paper. If your sight is normal you will see all the lines, if not, part of the graph paper will be blurred. Patchy loss of vision may be due to glaucoma (Chapter 8).

14

Migraine sufferers may also lose parts of the field of vision, but the attacks are usually limited to about half an hour (Chapter 11).

Half vision   Loss of half the field of vision may happen to one or both eyes. When the loss is in one eye the defective area may be either the upper or lower half, or the left or right half.

Occasionally the loss may be limited to a small segment or even to a quarter circle as, for example, in the section on a clock face from 12 to 3. When the trouble affects both eyes and lasts for up to half an hour migraine is probably the cause (Chapter 11). If the loss is more long-lasting it is likely to be due to a stroke or a brain tumour. Segmental loss of vision in one eye is due to blockage of blood vessels in the retina (Chapter 11).

Double vision   This is often confused with generalized blurred vision. The appearance of ghosting around something is not double vision, but if you see two objects instead of one you have double vision. You can be certain you have it if one object disappears when you close one eye.

The doubling may produce two images side by side, or one above the other. Occasionally one image may also appear to be leaning to one side.

Double or even triple vision can occur with early cataracts, but this of course will be seen with the affected eye only. True double vision can occur with high blood pressure, diabetes, strokes and multiple sclerosis (Chapter 11).

Flashing lights and spots   Flashes of light like sparks or zigzag lightning occur in migraine (Chapter 11). These last about half an hour, but if they persist for longer you may have problems in your retina (Chapter 10). While migraine symptoms may occur in one or both eyes, only one of your eyes will be affected if these symptoms are caused by retinal troubles.

Occasionally black spots or streaks accompanied by flashes of light may be seen due to bleeding. These differ from the common small spots or floaters that everyone sees from time to time by being more dense and numerous. They may occur with high blood pressure or diabetes (Chapter 11) or retinal tears or detachment (Chapter 10).

Discomfort or pain

Eye strain   You sometimes notice a feeling of discomfort in or around your eyes when you are using your eyes – for reading, for example – if you have a focusing error for which you need glasses (Chapter 5) or if there is an imbalance between the muscles of your eyes (Chapter 7). The feeling sometimes begins when you wake up. Some people describe it as a pulling sensation behind their eyes. This may develop into a headache which seems to be between and behind both eyes. This feeling does not mean that you have done any real damage to your eyes such as you would have in straining a ligament. It is a sensation that goes away with rest and the correct treatment.

Pain   It is often very difficult to say exactly where the pain is coming from, either in, on or around your eye. Three main types of pain exist:

1. Superficial pain on the eye
2. Deep pain in the eye
3. Spreading pain.

Superficial pain may be gritty or sharp, like getting a piece of sand in your eye. Alternatively it may be the burning or stinging sensation that you get from peeling onions or smoke. This can happen when your eyes do not produce enough tears, or if you have conjunctivitis (Chapter 6). Superficial pain may also accompany hay fever irritation (Chapter 6).
   Deep pain can vary from a slight ache within or behind the eye with iritis (Chapter 6) to the very severe pain of acute glaucoma (Chapter 8). The pain is caused by spasm of the muscles that control the movement of the coloured iris and the size of your pupils.
   Spreading pain can be caused by many eye conditions, including iritis and other inflammatory conditions of the eye, but often is a symptom of more general illness. The pain may spread to your cheek, forehead, temple or the top of your head. Pain on top of your head that seems to have spread from the back of your head is usually due to neck problems and not your eyes. Pain around your eyes, forehead or cheek that is associated with tenderness is usually due to sinusitis and becomes throbbing and more painful if you bend down.
   Pain on one side of your forehead can indicate neuralgia or may be the first hint of shingles.

Headache   Although your eyes are commonly thought to be the cause for headaches, in the majority of cases they cannot be blamed; in fact it is often the other way round, and the spreading pain of a bad headache affects your eyes.

Discharge from your eyes
There are two types of discharge that can occur, watery or sticky.

Watery discharge   The commonest form is the excess tears you produce if you get something in your eyes (Chapter 10). Alternatively, tears may overflow on to your cheeks because the normal drainage channels into your nose are blocked (Chapter 6).
   A watery discharge may also be caused by a virus infection, in which case the eye is also red (Chapter 6).

Sticky discharge You will be used to finding some crusting on your eyelids when you wake in the morning. This tends to collects on the edges of the lids beside the nose and is made up of salts left after tears have evaporated. But if you have a yellowish discharge of pus, particularly when you wake up, you have conjunctivitis (Chapter 6).

A sticky discharge with strings of mucus can indicate that your eye is dry through insufficient tears (Chapter 6).

Altered appearance of your eyes

Changes in the appearance of your eyes are usually due either to distortion of your eyelids or to a change in your eyeball.

The lids Swelling of the eyelids can result from a stye or chalazion (Chapter 6). These cause considerable distension of the skin and sometimes the eye is completely shut. The swelling can also spread across the bridge of the nose to affect the other side of the face.

The upper eyelid may droop down on one or both sides due to weakness of the muscles that keep the eyes open. This can happen to children who have the condition ptosis (Chapter 7), or to elderly people as a normal ageing change. A sudden drooping of the upper eyelid in an adult may happen with a stroke or brain tumour (Chapter 11). The lower eyelids may turn outwards in elderly people as the muscles of the lids become slack (Chapter 6).

The eyeball Alteration of the position of the eyes is commonly seen with a squint. One eye usually turns inwards though it may, less often, turn outwards (Chapter 7). The eyeball may appear pushed forwards and very large in short-sighted people (Chapter 5) and it may also be prominent in disease of the thyroid gland (Chapter 11).

A redness of the white of the eye can happen with many diseases (Chapter 6). Occasionally there may be a yellowish appearance if you have jaundice, or greyish colour as part of an ageing change.

From this summary you can see that many eye problems have the same symptoms. Correct diagnosis at an early stage is obviously most important and you should not hesitate to go for a test if you have any of the symptoms I describe. In the next chapter I talk about the tests a doctor or eye specialist may make to the different parts of your eye, according to your symptoms.

3 HOW YOUR EYES ARE EXAMINED

When you start to notice eye trouble, such as I described in Chapter 2, you will need to have your eyes examined by someone who is qualified and who has the proper instruments. You should make an appointment either with your family doctor or, for a sight test, an optician or optometrist. If after the first testing your doctor thinks you should see a specialist you will be recommended to see an ophthalmologist at the local hospital, or to a special eye clinic.

You may be confused by all the different terms used for the people who treat your eyes. Here are some guidelines to those you may see.

An ophthalmologist is a medically qualified doctor who has specialized in eyes. Only he or she is trained to diagnose and treat all eye problems. The term ophthalmic surgeon is also used.

An optician or optometrist is a person who has been trained to examine your eyes for focusing errors, to recognize diseases and to prescribe glasses or contact lenses. He or she cannot treat diseases except to give exercises for weak eye muscles. If an optician suspects an eye disease, you are referred to an ophthalmologist for treatment. The role of the optician or optometrist is important in detecting disease during the usual glasses test.

In the United Kingdom there are two types of opticians. Ophthalmic opticians test for focusing errors and prescribe and dispense (sell) the appropriate glasses or contact lenses. A dispensing optician only dispenses the prescribed glasses.

In North America, the name optometrist is given to someone trained in the same way as an ophthalmic optician in the United Kingdom. To confuse the issue, the title Doctor is used by optometrists.

Orthoptist This term is used for someone who has been trained to examine and manage squints and to carry out treatment under the supervision of an ophthalmologist (see also Chapter 7).

Oculist This is the all-embracing term for anyone who provides eye treatment.

When to have your eyes examined

It is sensible for you to get advice about your eyes if you develop any of the following symptoms (see also Chapter 2 for a more detailed description of symptoms):

- A worsening of your vision
- An alteration in the appearance of your eyes such as swelling of a lid or redness of the white of the eye
- Discharge from your eyes
- Pain.

You may be one of those people who dread having their eyes examined more than going to the dentist. This is probably because fear of the unknown applies more to the eyes than to any other part of the body, and because of their extreme sensitivity. However, the major part of the examination can be performed without your eyes even being touched. When it is necessary to handle your eyes your doctor will use local anaesthetic eyedrops so that you have no pain.

The examinations needed to diagnose your problem will be:

1. For distance and near focusing
2. The outside of your eye
3. The inside of your eye.

Testing your vision

This test will be done for the commonest eye problems of long or short sight and astigmatism (see Chapter 5), for which glasses or contact lenses are prescribed, and it is the first test in the diagnosis of the more serious disorders of glaucoma, cataract and detached retina which I describe in Chapters 8, 9 and 10.

Distance vision

This test assesses your long-distance vision. You are asked to read letters of decreasing size on a chart placed 20 ft (6 m) in front of you; alternatively, as a space-saving measure, a chart with the letters reversed is placed behind your head while you look in a mirror 10 ft (3 m) away. Although this may seem closer, in fact the distance is also 20 ft (6 m) from the letters to the mirror and back to your eyes.

Even though the chart is set at only 20 ft (6 m), the test measures your vision for that distance and for any point beyond it. Therefore, if you already wear glasses, use those that have been ordered for out-of-door use or for watching television. Do not think that because you are asked to read letters on the chart you should be wearing reading glasses.

Your doctor will cover one eye at a time and ask you to read down to the smallest letters that you can see. It is important to attempt the lowest line you can see even if you cannot clearly define every letter.

Normal vision is known as 6/6 in the UK or 20/20 in North America, meaning you can read all the letters of the bottom line at 6 m (20 ft). If you can read only the largest letter (on the top line) your vision is recorded as 6/60 or 20/200. This means that at 6 m (20 ft) you can only read a letter that would be seen by a normal sighted person at 60 m (200 ft). So, according to the number of lines you can read below the top one, you are given a rating.

Near vision

Your near vision is tested by reading a piece of print of differing sizes. This will be held at the distance normal to the particular occupation for which you need glasses. The usual distance is about 18 in (0.5 m), which is the average for reading at a desk. For reading a newspaper it may be slightly greater, while for needlework the focus is shortened and the sewing held at 10–12 in (25–30 cm).

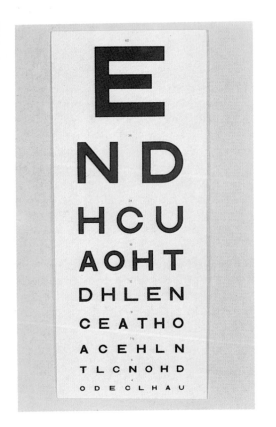

Normal-sighted people can read down to one line from the bottom of the chart, but some people can even see the lowest line.

If because of your work you have to be able to focus both at a particular distance and close to, you should tell your doctor. For example, a violinist must be able to see clearly the conductor and the music score, and a secretary will need to focus both on the desk and the typewriter.

If you have been tested by your doctor and have found difficulty with either distance or near vision tests he or she will suggest that you see an optician or optometrist who will decide if you need to wear glasses for the first time or if a change of your present pair is needed (see Chapter 4). An optician or optometrist can arrange new or altered glasses for you directly.

Field of vision test

What you see on either side of you while you are looking straight ahead is called your peripheral vision and this can be affected in cases of glaucoma, stroke or brain tumours. It is therefore the normal procedure for an optician or optometrist to check your field of vision at the same time as giving you the distance vision test if one of these problems is suspected. Certain drug treatments may also affect your field of vision (see Chapter 4).

Testing your own field of vision If you become aware that there is a worsening of your vision you can check your field of vision yourself. It will certainly be useful to tell the optician what you have discovered, but don't think it will be a substitute for the optician's examination.

1. Shut or cover your left eye and stare straight ahead at a point on a wall with your right eye. Hold your right hand about 1 ft (30 cm) away from your right ear over your shoulder. Gradually move your hand forward, at the same time moving your fingers. While looking straight ahead you will become aware of the movement at the edge of your vision.
2. Repeat this manoeuvre, bringing your hand up from your waist, down from above your head and across from your left-hand side.
3. You will find that you can see farthest out to your right-hand side and below, while the view to the left and above is restricted. This is because your nose and eyebrow limit the vision in these directions.

If in any of these manoeuvres you cannot see your moving fingers until you bring them directly in front of you, you have lost your peripheral vision. If your field of vision is normal the only point where your moving fingers will not be visible is in the area called the blind spot. This corresponds to a part of the back of the eye where there is no retina and where the optic nerve is formed. You can, for amusement, find you own blind spots using the diagram on page 22.

Close your left eye and look at the cross with your right eye. Gradually bring the book towards you and you will notice that the black spot disappears when the book is about 12 in (30 cm) away.

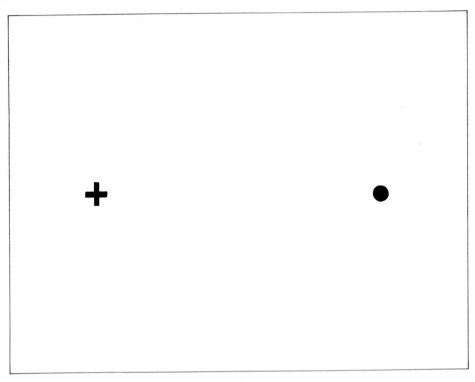

The blind spot test: see page 21 for instructions.

If you close your right eye and stare at the black spot with your left eye, the cross will disappear at the same distance.

Testing by a specialist The specialist's methods of testing your fields of vision check the same areas but with much greater accuracy.

In the commonest test you will be asked to watch a central point on a black screen while a white spot on the end of a wand is moved across the screen. Your field of vision is judged by you telling the specialist when the moving spot appears and disappears. Unfortunately, you will be tempted to follow the moving target rather than watch the central point, and so this test requires a lot of concentration on your part. It also has the disadvantage that the whole of the visual field cannot be assessed. However, this does not need testing except for rare conditions which if suspected will be tested by a further examination with a more complex machine.

A test that can be performed by non-medical assistants and so is often done at an optician's or optometrist's uses a screen on which a number of small spots light up. While looking at a central target you will be asked to say how many lights are visible. By adjusting the position and intensity of the lights an accurate measurement of your visual field can be made.

If you go for hospital tests it is possible that other, more complicated instruments will be used to examine your field of vision, but these are based on the same principles as the tests already mentioned.

Testing the eye muscles
The examiner will check how well your eyes work together by testing the movements of the eye muscles. This will show whether you have a squint or a tendency to squint (see Chapter 7).

Examining the outside of your eye
Your doctor needs to examine the outside of your eyes in order to be able to diagnose conditions that affect:

1. The lids, such as styes or ingrowing eyelashes
2. The white of the eye for conjunctivitis
3. The clear window or cornea for abrasions or ulcers.

The examination of the outside of your eye will usually be carried out using an adjustable reading light or a pen torch. Your doctor may also use a magnifying glass to see some of the small details of your eye.

The slit-lamp microscope is used to examine the finer details of the eye.

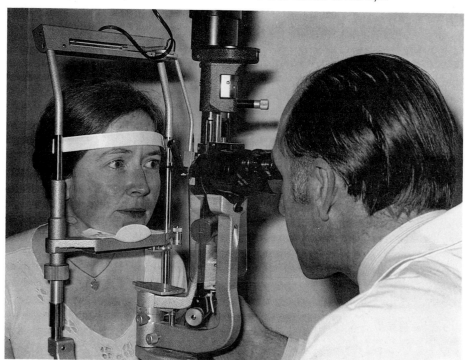

When you go to see an eye specialist you will be examined with a more complicated instrument called a slit-lamp microscope. This shows the specialist the fine detail of the front of the eye without discomfort to you.

Examining the inside of your eye
This will tell your doctor if you have any illness that affects:

1. The lens, such as a cataract
2. The light-sensitive retina, suggesting a general illness like diabetes or high blood pressure
3. The optic disc, for other disorders including glaucoma.

Your family doctor will examine you with an ophthalmoscope. This special type of torch allows the doctor to shine a light into your eye and to see the details of the lens and retina.

The ophthalmoscope has to be held very close both to the doctor's and your head, but again the procedure is quite painless. To look at the edge of the retina your doctor will ask you to look in various directions and it will help if you keep your head still and only move your eyes.

In order to get an even better view of your retina you may have eyedrops put in to enlarge your pupils. These take between fifteen and thirty minutes to act, during which time you may notice some blurring of your vision, especially for close focusing. Although it is possible to reverse the effect of the enlargement of the pupils with another type of eyedrop, some blurring may remain for a few hours. Because of this it is wise not to drive yourself home after the examination.

If your family doctor decides from this examination that you may be suffering from a problem such as diabetes or a detached retina (see Chapters 10 and 11), you will be recommended to see a specialist and given a more detailed test which will show up even the extreme edges of your retina.

After dilating your pupil, the specialist will instil a local anaesthetic eyedrop to numb the eye and you will be sat comfortably at a microscope. A special form of contact lens will be held against your cornea. This contains a series of mirrors set at different angles to show the retina. The test takes only a few minutes but you will find that your vision is slightly blurred because of the eyedrops and so, again, you should not drive.

Photography of the eye
Your ophthalmologist may want to record the appearance of your eyes so that comparisons can be made at future visits to see if there have been any changes in your condition. Photographs of the outer eye will be taken with an ordinary camera mounted on the examining microscope. When it is necessary to photograph the inside of your eye the pupil is dilated with eyedrops and more complex equipment is used.

A particular type of photography is needed for certain conditions that affect the retina, such as diabetes and this I describe in Chapter 11.

Colour blindness

Not everyone has normal colour vision. About one in twelve men and one in 250 women are colour blind. This is due to a defect that you are born with in the cells of your light-sensitive retina (see Chapter 1). The difficulties arise mainly with the colours red and green which are hard to distinguish and may appear grey. A very small minority confuse yellow and blue.

Testing for colour blindness

There is no treatment for colour blindness, but some jobs demand normal colour vision. For example, if you are applying to become a pilot, naval officer or train driver you will have to pass a test for colour vision. And if you want to be an electrician you will have to be able to distinguish the colour coding for electrical wiring. For anyone else, a degree of colour

The colour-blind test: the normal person can see the number 15 but if you see the number 17 you may be colour blind.

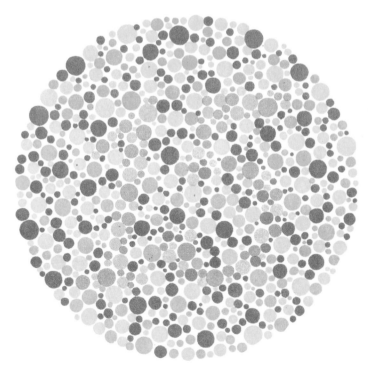

blindness is not likely to be a handicap. However, it can influence your ideas about looking at plants or paintings, or furnishing a room. So it is interesting to find out if your vision is normal. Try the test on page 25.

You are probably rather bewildered and possibly alarmed having read about all these tests that you may have to go through when you visit your doctor or specialist. However, as you will realize, none of them is painful, even if you have some discomfort and inconvenience when eyedrops are used.

The commonest test is of course to see if you need glasses and this I describe in more detail in Chapter 5. We must all eventually wear glasses to get our best vision. For most people this is just for reading, for others it may be to see clearly in the distance.

Before I describe the tests for and fitting of glasses, I will talk about everyday management of your eyes and the ways you treat them yourself for minor ailments.

4 HOW TO TREAT YOUR EYES

Your eyes are perfectly capable of looking after themselves for the greater part of your life. The seeing mechanism is protected by tissue and muscle and the eye generally kept in working order on the inside by the constant nutrition of the aqueous fluid and the outside by washing of the tears (see Chapter 1).

However, there are various disorders that I describe briefly in Chapter 2 which need specialist treatment; and for these you must go first to your doctor. I cannot recommend the patent medicines available over the counter as an alternative.

Treating normal eyes

Some people like to splash their eyes with cold water in the morning. If your eyelids are shut this certainly won't do any harm, or hurt them, but it won't do any good either, except to wake you up.

Cosmetic eyedrops, which claim to whiten the whites of your eyes and so make them sparkle, work well for some people, but there are always risks of allergic reactions. Make sure you are not getting sore eyes if you use this sort of drop, or you may end up with redder eyes than you had in the first place.

The use of an eye bath is not to be recommended. Your own tears do the job of washing the front of your eyes much better with each blink. You can get an abrasion on the front of your eye if the eye bath is mishandled and you may infect the eye with germs from a dirty eye bath; I think the term 'eye wash' is best kept for its slang derogatory meaning. If you want to get something out of your eyes, letting the tears wash it away or using a clean handkerchief are the best methods. I go into more detail on this in Chapter 10.

Cosmetics
Eye make-up is all right when applied in moderation and on the proper part of the eye. Some styles, though, are definitely harmful and I suggest you avoid doing any of the following:

- Wearing eyeliner inside the lashes, on the rims of the eyelids
- Wearing very thick mascara

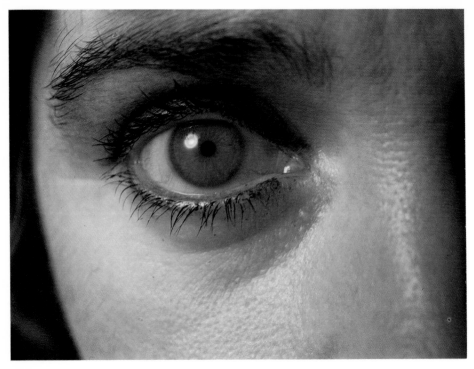

Wearing thick eye make-up inside the rims can make your eyes very sore.

- Wearing metallic-coloured eye shadow near the eyeball.
    In the first case the make-up is very likely to clog the tiny glands on the inside rim of your eyes which can irritate and may lead to an infection. In the case of mascara and metallic eye shadow, particles of the make-up fall on to your eyeball and stay there, building up in time to make for sore, red eyes.

Myths
These are some of the most common mistaken ideas about eyes and eyesight:

Glasses

- Wearing glasses does not weaken your eyes, neither does wearing the wrong ones.
- You do not strengthen your eyes by not wearing glasses when you really need them, you merely do not see so well.
- Just because you need to wear glasses doesn't mean you have weak eyes.
- Sunglasses are not bad for your sight.

Contact lenses

- Can't get displaced and lost behind your eyes.
- Wearing contact lenses does not prevent short sight from getting worse any more than putting a brick on a child's head stops him or her growing tall.

Lighting

- Too little light does not damage your sight, neither does too much, unless you stare at a very bright light, which may cause permanent damage.
- Fluorescent lighting does not strain your eyes.

Television

- Watching television does not damage your sight.
- There is no harm in sitting close to a television. Indeed some elderly people need to sit near the screen to see a large enough picture.
- It makes no difference to your eyes whether you have colour or black and white television.
- Visual display units on computers and word processors do not harm your eyes; neither does the light from photocopiers.

Exercises

- There are no exercises that will improve your sight. The only exercises that can be beneficial are those to strengthen the muscles that move your eyes from side to side (see Chapter 7).
- Rolling your eyes around has no effect, good or bad, on your sight.

Wearing your eyes out

- You cannot wear your eyes out by using them.
- Equally, you cannot preserve your sight by limiting your reading or close work.
- If the sight of one eye fails because of any disease, it does not throw any strain on the good eye or wear it out more quickly.

Squints

- You do not grow out of a squint.

Operations

- The eye is not taken out on to the cheek and then put back afterwards. It is attached by muscles and nerves that hold it in place.

Using eye treatments

Treatment for most eye problems is by eyedrops, ointment or occasionally by pills, depending on your particular problem and the condition of your eyes. In the chapters on the different disorders I shall explain which of the treatments is usual, and give the names of the drugs frequently prescribed (see Chapter 7 for giving treatment to children).

Eyedrops

These are easier to use than ointment and do not blur your sight as much. Here is the way to give them, either to yourself or to someone else:

1. Sit or stand with your head tilted backwards.
2. If you are right-handed, pull down the lower lid with the index finger of your left hand.
3. Hold the dropper bottle in your right hand. (If you are left-handed, pull the lid with your right-hand finger and hold the bottle with the left.)
4. Move the bottle in front of your eye with your bottle-holding hand resting on the other one.
5. Look to the top of your head and squeeze the bottle at the same moment. The drop will then fall on the less sensitive white of the eye. Do not touch the lids or the eyeball with the bottle. This will lessen the risk of later infection by the bottle.
6. Try to let the drop fall just inside the lower lid.
7. If you think that you have missed, put in another drop. It is impossible to put in too many drops as any excess will be blinked on to the lid margins and will run away.

   Because your tears – or any excess liquids – drain into your nose and on to the back of your tongue you may taste the drops after several minutes. Some eyedrops may sting, but this usually only lasts for a few seconds.

Because of their ingredients, some eyedrops should be stored in a cool place. This will be shown on the bottle. The best place is the refrigerator, providing you do not put the bottle in the ice compartment. Cool eyedrops are easier to put in as you can feel when the cold liquid is on your eye.

Ointment

This is more difficult to use than drops; it tends to blur your vision and it can make your eyelids and cheek greasy. The advantages of using an ointment are that it stays on the eye itself longer and is not diluted by tears in the same way as eyedrops, and so the drug in the ointment will have more chance to do its work. In one particular case, that of atropine, it is always wise to give the drug to babies in an ointment as with drops they may absorb too much in their bodies.

This is the right way to apply ointment:

1. If the tube needs to be kept cool because of its ingredients the ointment will thicken. Warm the tube for a few minutes and you will find it much easier to use.
2. Using a mirror, pull down the lower lid with the index finger of your left hand if you are right-handed (use your right hand if you are left-handed).
3. Hold the tube in your other hand.
4. Squeeze out about ¼ in (5 mm) of ointment into the inside of the lower lid.
5. If the ointment tends to remain on the nozzle rather than the eye, close your lids to cut off the ointment from the tube; don't worry about the tip of the tube touching your lids – this is something you can't avoid.
6. Massage the eye gently to distribute the ointment and wipe any excess off the lids with a clean paper tissue.

Keep to your treatment
Whether you are prescribed eyedrops, ointments or pills, you need to follow some basic rules to make sure you get the full benefit.

1. Make sure you know how frequently your doctor wants you to have the treatment, and for how long, and follow the instructions on the label carefully.
2. Try to even out the intervals between doses. If you are told to use eyedrops three times each day, leave eight hours between each treatment. It is no good taking three doses before lunch and then having no treatment until the following morning. This is particularly important in the treatment of glaucoma (Chapter 8).
3. If you need, say, three doses each day, do not double the dose, assuming that it will be twice as effective!
4. Never use eyedrops or ointment that have been prescribed for someone else.
5. Throw away eyedrops and ointment that have been opened for twenty-eight days as the preservatives may no longer be effective.

Allergy to treatment
One final point about these treatments: it is quite possible that you may be allergic to eyedrops, ointment or tablets. Allergy to drops or ointments tends to be more common in those who have an allergic tendency with asthma or the skin rash, eczema. Allergy to eye treatments is rare but it can affect the young or the old.

You may become allergic to a particular drug when it is first prescribed or the trouble may develop later even though at first you had no problems.

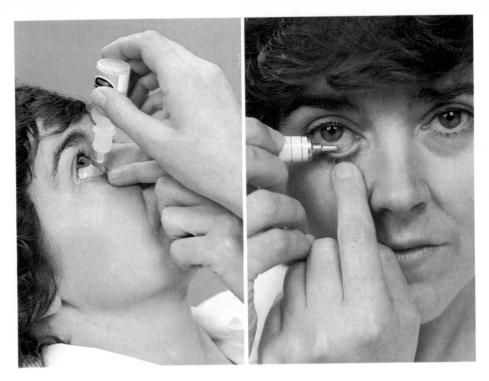

The correct ways of putting in eyedrops, *left*, and ointment, *right*.

Such allergies develop to the drug in the eyedrop or ointment. One example is a reaction to the antibiotic neomycin used for infections such as conjunctivitis or to the drug atropine used to dilate your pupils. Occasionally people become sensitive to the preservative in the eyedrop solution, or to the cream that is used in eye ointments.

If you are allergic to the treatment your eyes will become red and begin to itch within a few hours of using it. Your eyelids become puffy and may be so swollen that your eyes are difficult to open. The skin tends to wrinkle and may become moist. However, the trouble looks more serious than it really is, and will usually settle within a few days once the treatment has been stopped. The swelling of your lids due to fluid may involve your cheeks too. Because of gravity it tends to spread downwards and you may get a puffiness under your chin. Your doctor can give you either eyedrops or pills to help damp down the irritation and redness.

The skin of the lids may become flaky as the trouble settles, but eventually it will return to normal.

5 GLASSES AND CONTACT LENSES

The most common eye problems are to do with focusing. For these the remedy is to wear glasses or contact lenses to adjust your focusing to the required distance.

The focusing problems

In Chapter 1 I explained how the normal eye focuses on near and far objects by the ciliary muscle altering the focusing power of the lens. However, there are several cases when this mechanism doesn't work successfully:

1. You will be short-sighted if you have a long eye
2. You will be long-sighted if you have a short eye
3. You will have astigmatism if your eye is irregularly shaped
4. As you grow older the ciliary muscle works less effectively and you can't focus on close objects. This is called presbyopia.

What is short sight?
In short sight, or myopia, the objects that are far away appear blurred and it is only possible to see near objects clearly. The worse the short sight the closer the object must be placed.

Short sight is usually due to the eyeball being longer than normal and is an inherited characteristic. The image is formed in front of the retina and as it is impossible for the lens to move the position of the image back as far as the retina, glasses are needed to alter the focus and so allow distance vision.

For close vision such as reading, the myopic person can either accommodate to focus on the print or remove his or her glasses and use the short-sighted focus, bringing the object up close.

Another cause of short sight is linked with old age, when it is produced by changes within the lens of the eye. This I shall discuss in Chapter 9.

What is long sight?
In long sight, or hypermetropia, it is possible for the young person to see clearly without glasses both in the distance and for reading. With increasing age, the long-sighted person may require glasses for both distances.

The long-sighted eye is shorter in length than normal so that the image is formed behind the retina. As in myopia, this can be an inherited characteristic.

Before the age of forty the lens of your eye is able to alter the position of the image so that distant objects become clear. By further refocusing the eye can also be made to see nearby objects. This is why the young long-sighted person can manage without glasses. However, with increasing age the muscles in your eye are less active and so it becomes more difficult to alter the focus (see page 9). Glasses will be needed for reading and eventually for distance vision.

It is this need for distance glasses that tends to shock the middle-aged long-sighted person who has always had excellent distance vision and is suddenly faced with the need for both distance and reading glasses.

What is astigmatism?
This error of focusing of the eye is more complex than long or short sight. Its cause is a distorted lens system that you are born with; this can be an inherited condition. The shape of the lens or cornea is rather like the back of a spoon, where the curve along the bowl is longer than the curve across.

Short sight, *above*, and long sight, *below*, and how they are corrected.

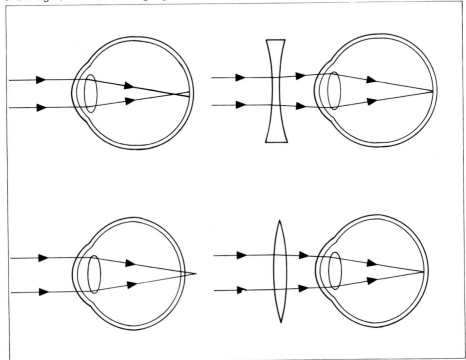

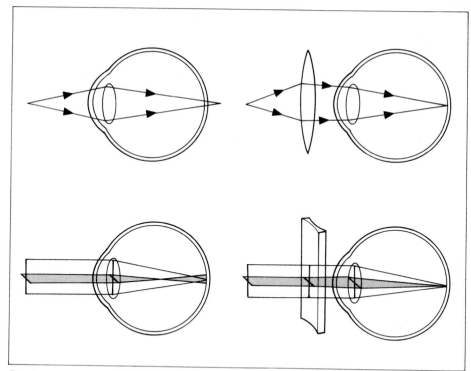

Presbyopia, *above*, and astigmatism, *below*, uncorrected and corrected.

So, in astigmatism the position of the image varies depending on the angle that light enters the eye. If a vertical beam or sheet of light enters the eye and can be sharply focused on the retina, a horizontal beam is focused in the same eye in front of the retina (see the diagram above).

It is not possible for the eye to refocus to correct astigmatism, but fortunately the error can be corrected with lenses which are cylindrical in shape.

What is presbyopia?

The closest position that you can hold a book and still see it clearly is called the near point. In children or short-sighted people this may be as close as 3 or 4 in (8 or 10 cm). With increasing age the lens of the eye hardens and the ciliary muscle weakens and so you are unable to change the focus so easily. This results in the near point gradually receding so that a book has to be pushed farther away while the head is held back. Eventually the near point reaches beyond arm's length and reading glasses are needed. This change is called presbyopia.

It is very gradual so that at first you will find only that you have to hold the book in a brighter light in order to see clearly. Usually by the age of forty or forty-five glasses become necessary for close work.

This change is often the first sign of approaching middle age and as a result of course you may be reluctant to admit that you cannot see and so may not want to wear glasses. Some people believe that glasses will further weaken their eyes and prefer to soldier on without them. I can assure you that it does not follow that the more you wear glasses the more you will need to wear them, and that it is not true that they will weaken your eyes. Equally mistaken is the widely held belief that by not wearing reading glasses and/or doing 'eye exercises' you can strengthen your eyes (see page 29).

Reading glasses become an essential optical prop to lean on. With them you can read, without you cannot. So it makes good sense to wear them when the need arises.

Testing for glasses or contact lenses

If you think you may need glasses try this simple test. Try to read the print on a newspaper at about 20 ft (6 m). You will probably manage the large headlines easily, but it becomes increasingly difficult with the smaller print. Now punch a small hole with the tip of a ball-point pen in a piece of card. Look through the hole at the newspaper with one eye while closing the other. If you read more clearly through the hole in the card than without, then it is worthwhile getting your eyes checked to see if you need glasses.

If you already wear glasses or contact lenses make sure you have your sight tested every two years. Regular testing is necessary as your vision can get worse very gradually, so that you may not notice it yourself.

Don't forget to take your most recent pair of glasses or contact lenses with you. This may seem an obvious point, but it is amazing how many people come for an eye examination without them!

You may have your eyes tested either by an ophthalmologist, or an optician, or an optometrist. A lot of people choose to be tested at an optician's or optometrist's as they can get the glasses or contact lenses there too.

Refraction
The first test you will be given is called refraction. This is to find out which, if any, focusing errors you have. Essentially, your specialist will judge what sort of lens you need by shining a light into your eye and watching its reflection. There are now several sophisticated instruments that can do this job automatically. You look into the instrument and the electronic equipment measures your focusing. They may look impressive but do not assume that they are necessary to carry out the best test. While

they may make the specialist's task easier, they do not guarantee that the glasses ordered for you will be any more accurate.

The distance vision test
From the results of the refraction test the optician can select the appropriate lenses for you. These will be put either into a special frame that you wear like glasses or into an instrument you look through. You will then be asked to read the letters on the distance vision chart (see page 20) and by making changes in the power of the lenses the optician or optometrist will gradually achieve your best vision.

This test often makes people very flustered. They feel that they must make an instant decision when asked to judge the difference between two lenses. Don't let yourself be hurried. If you aren't sure which lens gives the clearest vision, ask your specialist if you can try both lenses again.

Near vision
When you have reached your best distance vision the specialist will check your near vision. You may find the distance correction has also improved the near vision satisfactorily. It is more likely after the age of forty-five that a further adjustment to the power of the lenses will be necessary. In any case make sure that your optician knows what you need your near vision for most, to read, for work, or to do needlework, for example.

Testing for contact lenses
The above tests will all be made whether you are going to use glasses or contact lenses. The strength of the contact lenses is calculated by the specialist from the strength of ordinary lenses assessed for you and some measurements are taken to judge the exact shape and size of your cornea.

Glasses

Choosing the frames
After the specialist has decided which lenses you need the prescription will be made up for you. But first, if you want to wear glasses you will need to choose suitable frames, and for this you must go to an optician's or optometrist's, whether you were tested there or by an ophthalmologist. The choice that you make will be influenced by a number of things: the use of the glasses and their appearance are the most important, while the cost must often be taken into consideration.

There is a wide selection of frames made from metal, plastic or a combination of the two. Although we all have definite ideas about how we would like to look, choosing the right frame can be difficult. It may help to take your partner or a friend, but in the end it is wisest to be guided by your optician, who will know from the large selection which frame is most likely to suit you, both from a cosmetic and a practical point of view. Very large frames may be fashionable but they may not be practical if you need thick lenses, while thick frames may act as blinkers and restrict your side vision for certain occupations such as driving.

To help you make your choice, here are a few facts about different types of frames.

1. Metal frames can be straightened if they become misshapen, while plastic frames tend to break more easily.
2. In rimless frames the lenses are held in place by nylon cord or screws. They have the advantage that no frame is visible, especially when you look down.
3. Glasses have either a saddle bridge or two pads supporting the weight on either side of the nose. If you need glasses with heavy lenses a saddle bridge is the better choice as it distributes the weight evenly over the bridge of the nose. The two pads can be uncomfortable and are likely to bend out of place.
4. Some people who suffer from allergies may develop a skin rash from metal frames, particularly those made from nickel.
5. Children and anyone playing sport will be helped by ear pieces that curl around the back of the ears and keep the frames firmly in place.

Lenses

There are a number of important points to consider when you choose your lenses. You need to think about your occupation and lifestyle when deciding the material and type of lens you want. Again, your optician or optometrist should help you.

Glass or plastic?   Lenses are made either of glass or plastic. Glass has the advantage of being more difficult to scratch, but it is heavier. It can break easily, producing dangerous splinters that can harm the eyes. It is possible to toughen glass when it is made which reduces this risk, but it does not remove it entirely.

In contrast, plastic is light but tends to scratch. It is the ideal material for sport because of the safety aspect. Plastic lenses also tend to mist over less than glass when you go from a cold atmosphere into warm surroundings.

Half lenses   If you need glasses for close work but not for distance and have to alter your focus a lot, for example, if you are sketching, half-moon shaped lenses may be the most useful. With them you can focus on distant objects as you look up, without having to take off your glasses.

However, you may not be happy with the appearance – perhaps the shape makes you look older – in which case bifocals are an alternative.

Bifocal lenses If you need glasses for distance and near vision, you should consider having bifocal or multifocal lenses. It is often inconvenient to have to keep changing glasses when you wish to read but need to use your distance vision as well. This can be overcome by using a bifocal lens, which has both the distance and reading segments in one lens. If you do not need a distance lens, as an alternative to the half glasses you can still have bifocals with the top of the lens made from plain glass and your reading lens at the bottom.

One of several different sizes of reading segment can be ordered, depending on your particular needs. This can vary from occupying the whole of the lower half of the lens to a small segment set just below the centre.

The commonest bifocal has a small area for near vision at the bottom of the distance vision lens. This offers the best solution for everyday use.

Another bifocal has a small reading segment surrounded by the distance lens. The small rim below allows you distance vision when looking down. This can be a help in negotiating steps, when you need your feet to be in focus.

Multifocal lenses Occasionally it is necessary to be able to focus sharply on an intermediate distance of, say, 6–10 ft (2–3 m). Most people are able to see clearly enough through the distance part of a bifocal lens. However, focusing at different distances gets more difficult as you get older and the ciliary muscle works less efficiently. If you cannot make these adjustments in focusing you can have another segment inserted to make a trifocal lens.

Alternatively the lens can be made so that there is a gradual change from distance vision at the top to near vision at the bottom. This sounds ideal but in practice these lenses do not suit a lot of people. There is only a small portion that produces a sharp image for each distance; and there may be some distortion when you turn to look through the edge of the lens.

When bifocal and multifocal lenses are generally unsuitable

1. They are no use if you wish to be able to look up and still see clearly at a close distance. For example, a librarian will be unable to read the book titles on a high shelf and a home decorator will have difficulty painting above eye level.
2. They should not be worn by anyone with neck problems. The constant tilting of the head up and down can aggravate arthritis.
3. They should not be worn if you suffer from unsteadiness or difficulty with walking because of the blur when you look down.
4. It is unwise to wear bifocals if your job involves working at heights or climbing ladders.
5. Your optician may advise against this type of lens if you have astigmatism because of the distortion effects.
6. If you wish to read in bed it is better to wear ordinary reading glasses

which save you from having to tilt your head backwards as you would with bifocals.

Tinted lenses Tinted lenses are becoming more and more popular. You may want them for cosmetic reasons, to reduce the glare of the sun, or there may be a genuine medical reason for reducing the amount of light reaching your eyes, for example, if you have cataracts. Remember, though, that your eyes work by light so that a reduction in light may result in a reduction in vision.

A tint may be either fixed or variable. A fixed tint is either incorporated in the lens material or added to the surface after the lens has been made. This means that you can have an old pair of your distance glasses tinted by your optician or optometrist to whatever colour you want. Some office workers reading under bright fluorescent lighting find that a very pale blue or grey is comfortable. People with cataracts prefer a darker tint.

Polaroid lenses, which are also a fixed tint, are especially effective in cutting out glare and so are useful when you are near water or snow. Don't forget that when you are driving they may produce an annoying patterning on the windscreen.

Variable or photochromic tints alter their density depending on the

Different types of bifocal and trifocal lenses.

40

amount of ultraviolet light: the brighter the light the darker their tint becomes. Several gradations and colours are available. The darkening process takes up to thirty seconds, but the bleaching so that the lens becomes lighter may take several minutes. This type of tinting can be used with glass lenses but not plastic ones. Variable-tint lenses can be unsuitable for driving as car windscreens can filter the available ultraviolet light so that the lens is not fully activated.

Are sunglasses necessary?

It is not possible to damage sight with the everyday light that we experience, even in the hottest climates – although you can of course permanently affect your vision if you are ever unwise enough to stare at the sun, regardless of whether it is rising, setting or even during an eclipse (see Chapter 10).

Sunglasses are restful, though, particularly for very fair people who suffer a lot from glare, and they will certainly not damage your eyes, as some people fear. It doesn't matter which sort you choose; but it is worth bearing these points in mind when you buy a pair:

1. Make sure the frames are comfortable as you'll be wearing them when it's hot.
2. Make sure the lenses show no distortion, especially at the centre, and that they cover your field of vision.
3. For everyday wear the colour of the lenses and whether they are fixed or variable is a matter only of choice and cost. Some lenses are designed for maximum protection against harmful wavelengths and these are useful for skiers and airplane pilots.
4. If you have severe light sensivity you should consult an optician or optometrist.

Contact lenses

Having contact lenses fitted is an alternative to wearing glasses to correct your distance vision. But they can never be a substitute for reading glasses. If you need to wear reading as well as distance glasses you will still need to wear the reading glasses over your contact lenses for near focusing.

Contact lenses are most commonly worn to correct short sight; they can also be used for long sight and astigmatism. But they are not suitable for everyone. I would not recommend them for you:

1. If you are at all squeamish about your eyes.
2. People who are clumsy with their hands, as they may harm their eyes while putting the lenses in or taking them out.
3. If you work in particularly dusty or dirty conditions where particles could easily get behind the lenses.

4. If you have an allergic condition such as hay fever which makes your eyes itchy.

But most people who have worn contact lenses successfully never want to return to glasses except for reading. Vision is often better than with glasses, and as the lenses move with your eyes there is no distortion on looking to the side such as you get with glasses with thick lenses. Contact lenses do not mist in a warm room or get wet in the rain as glasses do.

Types of contact lens

Contact lenses are described as either hard or soft. The terms refer to the consistency of the materials that are used to make the lenses.

Hard lenses   These are made of hard plastic and are a little smaller than the cornea. They stand up well to everyday wear and tear, but because of their hardness have certain drawbacks. You have to get used to them by building up a tolerance to them over several weeks. Starting two hours each day for several days, you gradually increase by half an hour the length of time you wear the lenses until you are able to tolerate them all day. You cannot expect your eyes to cope immediately with hard lenses any more than you would expect to be able to walk all day wearing a new pair of heavy boots. But the feeling of discomfort as if you had a foreign body in your eye, which of course it is, disappears remarkably quickly.

A hard lens prevents the cornea from getting the oxygen from the air and so the eye may become sore. For people with this problem the gas-permeable lens is a suitable common alternative. Although this is a hard lens the material allows oxygen to reach the cornea.

Soft lenses   These are made of a pliable material that absorbs water like a sponge. The lens is larger than a hard lens and may be bigger than the cornea so that the edge rests on the white of the eye. Despite being bigger it is more comfortable to wear and because of its water content oxygen can reach the cornea more easily. There is no need to build up a tolerance gradually in the way that you have to with hard lenses.

Like hard lenses, soft ones are only worn during the daytime and removed before you go to sleep. One type of soft contact lens can be worn constantly, only being changed about every six to eight weeks. However I prescribe this type of lens only for patients who have had cataract surgery as people wearing them need to be kept under close supervision. The risks of infection and breakage make them less suitable for regular use, although some people wear them satisfactorily.

What are the disadvantages of soft lenses?

1. If you have marked astigmatism your vision may not be as sharp as with hard lenses.

42

2. Because the lens material is soft it can crack or even break more easily, so that soft lenses need to be replaced more often.
3. They may become covered by spots of mucus and because of their sponge-like consistency are more difficult to keep clean. This problem with cleaning and sterilizing means that infection is more common with soft than with hard lenses.
4. The solutions used to clean and disinfect the lenses may also cause irritation to the eyes, so they have to be carefully rinsed after cleaning according to the optician's or optometrist's instructions.

Which type should you choose?

Whether you have hard or soft contact lenses will depend on your need, assessed by your optician or optometrist: if your eyes are not particularly sensitive and you need to wear the lenses all the time, the hard type will probably be recommended, as these give better vision. For anyone with very sensitive eyes who cannot get on with hard lenses, or who wishes to wear lenses only occasionally, the soft type are better.

Looking after your contact lenses

Because contact lenses are worn right on the eyeball they must be kept sterilized to avoid your eyes becoming infected. This means that when you are not wearing them they should be kept in one of the special sterilizing solutions that your optician will recommend.

How often you clean the lenses depends on whether they are soft or hard. You will be told exactly how and when your lenses need cleaning by your optician or optometrist.

When you are not wearing your lenses, keep them in their own container, so that they stay absolutely clean and you don't lose them.

Insurance

It certainly makes sense to insure both contact lenses (which are so easy to lose) and glasses against loss. You should get advice from your optician or insurance broker about this.

Although it may be a depressing thought that everyone at some time will need glasses or contact lenses, the very fact that they are so universally worn means they are constantly being improved in effectiveness, comfort and appearance. So we are far better off today than even fifty years ago. For a relatively low cost focusing problems in people of any age can be improved. Don't be too proud to admit you've got to the point when you need glasses, whatever your age. To anyone wondering when presbyopia will catch up with them, I offer the advice I give my patients: if your arms are too short for reading, it's time to have your eyes tested!

In the next chapter I shall be talking about other eye conditions that are likely to affect everybody at some time – in general the less serious and most easily treated problems.

6 THE RED EYE AND CORNEAL PROBLEMS

Everybody gets red-looking eyes sometimes, but you may be surprised at the number of possible causes and the widely varying degree of seriousness of the conditions. In this chapter I describe the most common forms of red eye and their treatment. Troubles of the cornea can sometimes be caused by a red eye too.

Wet and dry eyes

Wet eyes   Your eyes will be wet and may redden if there are too many tears. This may happen because your eyes produce more tears in an attempt to wash away something in your eye such as an eyelash or in response to an irritant like smoke or when peeling onions.

They may also water if there is a blockage of the normal draining of tears into your nose. This often happens when you have a cold. It is also common for elderly people to get slightly watery eyes. This is due to a narrowing of the tear ducts rather than to a blockage of the plumbing.

A watery eye often develops conjunctivitis (see page 46), when it will become red and sticky.

Your doctor will treat this blocking of the ducts with antibiotic eyedrops, and these may also help the watering. If they don't you will be recommended to see a specialist to have the tear ducts syringed. This is a minor and painless procedure which your specialist will do at your first visit. Anaesthetic eyedrops are used but your vision should be unaffected so that you may drive afterwards.

If it is impossible to syringe the tear ducts you may be offered an operation to form a new channel for your tears to drain into your nose. This is a major operation with about an 85 per cent chance of success, so if the watering is only slight you may prefer to continue mopping your eyes – your drainage will probably be adequate for your own comfort, unless in your job frequent mopping of your eyes is very inconvenient.

Dry eyes   This is potentially a far more serious condition as tears are needed to keep your cornea healthy and transparent.

Dry eyes are caused by the tear gland producing insufficient tears. This is not very common but tends to occur in old age when it balances out poor tear drainage, and so is not noticeable. People suffering from rheumatoid arthritis frequently have dry eyes and the condition may then be associated with a dry mouth.

If you have too few tears your eyes feel gritty and each blink is uncomfortable. Your vision becomes poor and your eyes look red. In an attempt to overcome the dryness more mucus is produced which causes a stringy discharge that collects inside your lower eyelids.

Your doctor will prescribe artificial tears in the form of eyedrops and these may be used as often as you want. They act as a lubricant to the front of the eyes. The following should also help relieve the discomfort due to dry eyes:

1. Reduce the dryness atmosphere caused by central heating by using a humidifier.
2. Do not drive with the car heater on, especially if it is at face level.
3. Do not sit in front of direct heat from a gas or electric fire.
4. Certain activities like watching television, reading or sewing may make your eyes more painful as you tend to blink less when concentrating, so use your eyedrops just before any of these occupations and remember to keep blinking regularly.

Examples of conjunctivitis: both eyes are usually red, sticky and gritty, and vision is blurred.

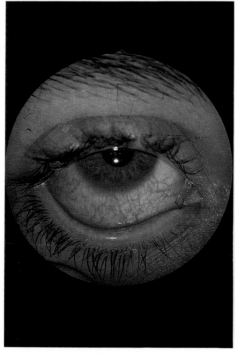
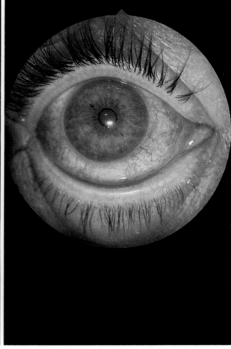

Conjunctivitis

Bacterial and viral conjunctivitis   This is probably the condition most commonly associated with the term 'red eye'. The strict meaning of this word is inflammation of the conjunctiva (the thin membrane covering your eyelids and sclera). However, popular usage has meant that most people apply it to the red sticky infected eye. This type of conjunctivitis is most commonly due to a bacterial infection being rubbed into the eyes from dirty hands or a soiled handkerchief, but viruses can also cause conjunctivitis – in which case it may be preceded by a cold or a sore throat. Viral conjunctivitis is commoner in adults than children, whereas bacterial conjunctivitis is very common in any age group, but especially in children.

Conjunctivitis usually affects both eyes, which become red with a sticky discharge so that your lids are glued together when you wake. Your eyes feel gritty and your vision is blurred.

Conjunctivitis can be catching and so you must take great care not to pass it on to someone else – you should not use anybody's towel but your own, nor rub your eyes with a borrowed handkerchief. Follow these rules to manage your own conjunctivitis:

1. Always wipe your eyes with a clean handkerchief.
2. If only one eye is affected make sure that you do not rub your eyes or wipe the normal eye with the same handkerchief.
3. Try to keep your hands as clean as possible, washing them well with soap and under a running tap (faucet).
4. Go to your family doctor to have a proper treatment prescribed for the condition. This will be eyedrops or ointment and you must follow the doctor's instructions conscientiously. You may have to use eyedrops as frequently as every hour during a very bad attack.
5. Do not stop the treatment as soon as the conjunctivitis appears to be settling but carry on for several days longer to make certain that all the infection has gone.

Viral conjunctivitis is difficult to treat as there is no known drug that is effective against the viruses responsible. The symptoms of viral conjunctivitis gradually settle over a few weeks but occasionally drag on for several months. Your doctor can help by prescribing eyedrops that will make your eyes more comfortable.

Allergic conjunctivitis   This common condition produces marked irritation of your eyes which become red and sometimes sticky due to infection.

You can be allergic to a large number of different things including house dust, pollen or pet animals. Irritation and swelling of your eyelids may accompany hay fever, wheezing or even asthma and the skin rash, eczema.

Your eye symptoms may occur all the year round with allergies to house dust and animals but tend to be seasonal when the cause is pollen. As with all allergies, this is a condition you are unlikely to be able to cure completely.

A particular form of allergic conjunctivitis called spring catarrh occurs in young children who suffer from asthma and eczema, and is more severe than the itchy eyes associated with hay fever.

There are several different eyedrops that your family doctor can prescribe to lessen the irritation of allergic conjunctivitis. One new drug that has proved successful is Opticrom. However, if none of these work your doctor will refer you for specialist treatment. Unfortunately injections to desensitize you will not help your eye symptoms as much as they will the wheezing.

The only practical measures you can take yourself are to keep away as much as possible from the things you are allergic to.

For example, if you are allergic to dust get your mattress vacuum cleaned frequently, or if feathers bother you, use foam pillows. Your doctor or specialist will no doubt be able to suggest many more practical ways of avoiding aggravating your allergic condition.

Allergies to drugs People can suddenly develop an allergy to a drug they have been prescribed for a particular condition and this may result in an allergic red eye, with reddened, puffed-up lids, weeping and crusting of the surrounding skin. Atropine and neomycin are examples of drugs that sometimes produce this allergy.

This must be the easiest allergy to treat: tell your doctor, who will take you off that drug.

Contact allergies Cosmetics, metal fasteners, dyes in clothes are only some of the items that can cause an itchy skin allergy called contact dermatitis. If you rub your eyes the condition can be transferred to your eyes, which will become red and itchy and swell up. So it is extremely important to avoid touching your eyes if you have a contact allergic condition.

Subconjunctival haemorrhage

As you get older your blood vessels become more fragile and in the elderly discoloration due to bleeding under the skin is quite common and happens without any injury. Something similar can happen to your eyes and could cause a bright red area which may spread to cover all of the white of the eye. It is painless and does not affect your vision. The blood is entirely on the outside of the eye and cannot get into your eye. It may occur at any time of day and may follow doing something strenuous. Alternatively it can happen at night and you first see it when you look in the mirror to shave or apply make-up.

No specific treatment is needed as the blood is gradually absorbed over a period of ten to fourteen days – although it may seem as though it isn't clearing at first because, being on the surface of your eye, the blood can readily absorb oxygen and stay bright red, unlike bruises which gradually change colour.

Very rarely, this happens repeatedly, and then the blood vessels in the eye can be sealed. But I would hardly ever recommend treatment for this mild condition.

Disorders of the white of the eye

Your eyes may become red with either of these two conditions. Pinguecula is a small yellowish swelling on the triangle of exposed white of the eye on either side of the clear cornea. It is common after the age of forty – in fact nearly everyone gets it at some time. Although it doesn't look very pleasant it does not affect the vision.

Pterygium is a fleshy swelling in the same position as a pinguecula but can interfere with your vision as it tends to grow across the surface of the cornea. This can affect anyone from the age of twenty onwards. It is rare and the cause is unknown, although it does occur more frequently in hot, dusty climates.

Eyedrops prescribed by your doctor can help redness of your eyes in either of these conditions. Surgical treatment is needed for a pterygium if it threatens your vision by growing across the line of sight. This is a minor procedure carried out under a local anaesthetic and you are treated as an outpatient. Occasionally the pterygium may regrow and require further surgery.

Corneal ulcers

Ulcers of the cornea are usually painful and all of them are potentially dangerous because of the risks to the sight. They may also give rise to iritis (see below).

An ulcer may be the result of:

- An injury such as you may get from a scratch from a twig in the garden or from bad handling of contact lenses. I go into more detail about this in Chapter 10.
- Infection arising from conjunctivitis.
- The virus herpes simplex which causes cold sores around your nose and mouth.

The virus is caught by direct contact so avoid being kissed by, or kissing anyone if you have a cold sore, especially on or near the eyes. Like cold sores on your lips, the ulcers in your eyes can recur: a head cold, being run down or under stress, sitting in a draught or too much sunlight can all trigger off a further ulcer.

Treatment   It is important to get treatment from your doctor as soon as possible to limit scarring. When the cause is an injury or an infection, as with conjunctivitis, your doctor will prescribe an antibiotic eyedrop. For viral ulcers there are several eyedrops available that will help to heal the ulcer, but with this sort you are always liable to a further attack (see above).

Corneal graft operations
This operation replaces an abnormal cornea with a disc of clear cornea taken from the eye of someone who has died. The disc can be up to ½ in (1 cm) in diameter and the same thickness as the affected cornea, when the operation is called a penetrating graft, or it may replace only the outermost layers of the cornea, when the operation is known as a lamellar graft. The grafted piece of cornea is kept in position by very fine nylon stitches.

When is a graft needed? The clear cornea may become cloudy as a result of disease or following injury:

1. Herpes simplex infection – the cold sore virus – can produce ulceration and scarring of the cornea. While the infection can be treated with antiviral drugs, if the scarring is severe a graft is needed.
2. A condition called keratoconus causes thinning and distortion of the cornea. This may also need a graft.
3. Occasionally because of an inherited defect.
4. The commonest worldwide cause of a cloudy cornea is trachoma. This is an infective disease found in countries where poverty, over-crowding, lack of sanitation and poor hygiene are common. The infection, caused by a virus-like organism, produces conjunctivitis, which in turn causes scarring and distortion of the eyelids.

The majority of corneal graft operations are successful. Since the cornea does not contain any blood vessels the chances of rejection are much lower in this than in other graft operations. However, rejection of a corneal graft does sometimes occur and then the disc of the new cornea becomes cloudy and opaque. Treatment by your specialist will help to reduce this.

After the operation
Your eye will be bandaged for about a week and you will have to keep fairly still, as after a cataract operation (see Chapter 9). You will be given eyedrops to use for at least a month.

For the first three or four weeks at home you should do only sedentary work and not take part in any vigorous sports for two to three months.

Donating your eyes
If you feel that you would like to restore someone else's sight after you have died you can donate your eyes so that your cornea can be used in a graft. Most eyes are suitable for a graft operation except those of the very

young or the very old. Some illnesses like infective hepatitis or leukaemia or eye ailments such as iritis or glaucoma also make them unsuitable. If you are uncertain about your eyes being usable for a graft you can find out from your doctor or local eye clinic whether it is worth being a donor.

Donating your eyes is similar to being a kidney donor and you can carry a donor card in the same way, so that in the case of an accident or sudden death your eyes may be used. But it is wise also to let your nearest relatives know of your intentions. It is all too easy for cards or signed papers to be forgotten in the crisis of a death. Relatives must inform the local eye hospital as soon as possible, preferably within a few hours, otherwise changes take place in the eyes which mean they cannot be used.

Iritis

This is an inflammation of the front half of your eye, particularly the coloured iris, and it usually affects only one eye. It is an uncommon condition. The muscles of the iris and lens go into spasm, causing a deep discomfort inside the eye and the white of the eye around the cornea becomes red. Bright lights hurt the eye and this may be first noticed when you are driving at night, with a stream of oncoming headlights making your eyes painful. One of my patients even noticed some soreness in his bad eye while lighting a cigarette. The condition develops usually within a day, and your vision becomes increasingly hazy.

In up to 60 per cent of cases there is no known cause for the disease. Occasionally it occurs as a complication of a more generalized illness, such as:

1. Rheumatoid arthritis, particularly in the form that affects children.
2. Iritis is a common complication if you develop a cold sore ulcer (herpes simplex virus), a corneal ulcer (see above), or if you get shingles affecting your forehead (herpes zoster virus).
3. The venereal infections of syphilis and gonorrhoea once easily treated by the antibiotic penicillin are now more common causes of iritis as they become resistant to antibiotic treatment.
4. Tuberculosis is now a rare cause of iritis but has been replaced by a widespread generalized condition called sarcoidosis which also affects the lungs but is not infectious like tuberculosis.

As with so many illnesses the sooner treatment is started the fewer complications you are likely to get. If you get the earliest symptoms such as discomfort, redness of your eye or blurring of your vision you should report to your doctor as soon as possible.

The doctor will usually refer you directly to a specialist if he or she suspects that you have iritis, because of the serious nature of the condition.

Treatment is with eyedrops that work against inflammation called corticosteroids. There are several sorts with differing strengths. You will also be given dilating drops to prevent the spasm and these may make your vision more blurred. If you are suffering from a lot of pain you will be given an analgesic.

Iritis tends to be a recurrent condition. The time between attacks can vary from weeks to months and occasionally it may be several years before you get any more trouble.

Disorders of the lids: styes

The commonest problem on the eyelids are styes. Everybody is liable to get a stye at some time, but more than likely it will be during childhood or the teenage years. The stye is an infection at the root of an eyelash commonly caused by the bacterium staphylococcus. It starts as a slight discomfort when you blink or touch the lids. Very quickly the lid becomes red and swollen around the eyelash that is affected. A small boil develops and eventually comes to a head and discharges. Like boils on other parts of the body, it is painful just before it discharges.

The old-fashioned remedy of rubbing a stye with a gold wedding ring has nothing to recommend it, and may even spread infection. Nothing needs to be done for the isolated stye. Some doctors suggest removing the affected eyelash but I think it is preferable to let it discharge on its own. Any pus can be wiped away with a clean paper tissue. You should not rub your eyes as you may transfer the infection to your healthy eye.

Repeated attacks of styes These may be due to various causes:

- Some children get crops of styes. This is usually the result of rubbing their eyes with dirty hands, especially if they have been playing with pet animals. If the child also has itchy eyes due to an allergy he or she may need treatment from a doctor, but otherwise common sense and cleanliness are usually enough.
- If you are in a low physical condition you will be susceptible to all sorts of infection including repeated styes.
- Styes are fairly common in people with diabetes.

You should see your doctor in the last two cases. He or she will give you antibiotic eyedrops to get rid of the infection and will test your urine to make sure that you do not have diabetes.

Chalazion

This swelling, also called a Meibomian cyst, occurs within the lid of one of the minute glands that normally produces an oily fluid. This fluid, which is part of the normal tear film, is spread over the eye by blinking. It helps delay the evaporation of your tears and prevents drying of your eye. The fluid, usually as a result of a conjunctival infection, can become too thick to escape from the gland, which then swells up. This produces a painless swelling under the lid, like a small half bead. The gland may become

51

infected and the lid becomes red, sore and swollen. Despite this a chalazion is not catching.

When a chalazion is small and painless it may disappear without any treatment over a period of six to eight weeks. However, if the chalazion will not go away but gets bigger and uncomfortable you should see your doctor. He or she may prescribe antibiotic eyedrops.

Alternatively, any acute discomfort can be eased by steam bathing. To do this cover a wooden spoon with some gauze or bandage. Dip the covered spoon into boiling water and then hold it so that with your head bent forward the steam can rise towards your eye. DO NOT TOUCH the lids with the spoon or you will burn them. When the spoon has cooled dip it into the water and repeat the process. The heat will act like a poultice on a boil by bringing the infection to a head so that it discharges. Steam bathing should be done for at least fifteen minutes twice a day.

When a chalazion is persistent it may grow so large that it will cause blurring of your vision. This is more common with a chalazion on the upper than on the lower lid, and is due to the lump pressing on your cornea so that your focus is affected. Your doctor will refer you to a specialist to have the chalazion opened. Under a local anaesthetic he will make a small cut on the inside of your lid to release the contents of the

A stye, *left*, is an infection in a lash root, while a chalazion, *right*, is a swelling in a gland of the eyelid.

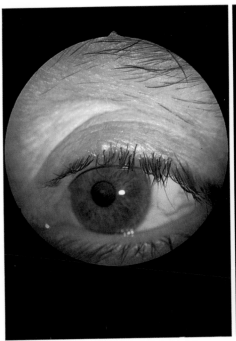
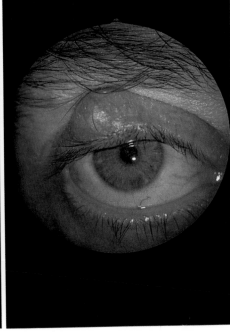

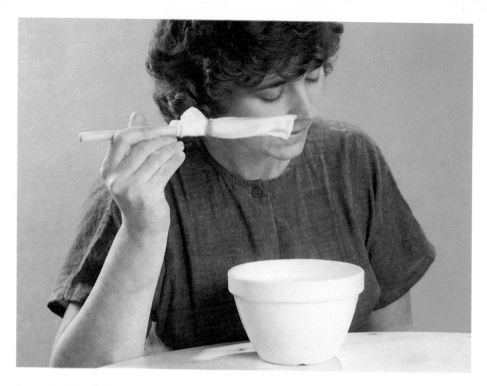

Steam bathing helps both styes and chalazions (see instructions opposite).

gland. Your eye will be padded for the rest of the day but you should be ready for work the following morning.

Even after this procedure there may still be a small swelling, especially if you have had the chalazion for several months or more but this will gradually disappear. You could compare the result to letting the air out of a football, with the oily secretion being the air and the wall of the gland the emptied football.

Blepharitis

Inflammation of the lids is called blepharitis. It can be due to various factors, from the sufferer having very fair and sensitive skin to a low-grade staphylococcal infection being caught.

The margins of the lids become red, so you look as if you have red, inflamed eyes, and dandruff-like scales stick to the eyelashes. This is an uncomfortable condition, making your eyes sore and gritty rather than painful. The inflammation can spread to the conjunctiva so that the eyeball looks red. Occasionally people get dandruff of the scalp and eyebrows at the same time as a blepharitis attack. Less often the lid edges become infected so that they have the appearance of being covered with multiple styes. But since the condition itself is an inflammation rather than an infection, blepharitis is not catching.

Blepharitis is a chronic problem which can affect anyone from the very young to the elderly. In fair, sensitive-skinned people, it is unlikely ever to disappear completely, although children can grow out of it. You can have episodes when an attack of blepharitis is severe and your eyes are very sore, but there are also times when you have no trouble at all.

Your doctor can prescribe a local antibiotic ointment or occasionally an anti-inflammatory drug as an ointment – this treatment will improve the condition but it cannot cure it. The ointment should be rubbed into the eyelash roots after you have removed the scales with damp cotton wool.

Distortion of the lids
These conditions are due to changes in the eyelid muscles, and cause redness and discomfort.

Ectropion   In the over-seventies it is common for the lower lids to turn outwards and cause slight watering of the eyes as the tears can't drain into the ducts in the normal way. This is known as ectropion.

Entropion,   that is, the lids turning inwards, occurs in the same age group and is also common. The lid turns in, due to the muscles going into spasm, and the eyelashes rub on the cornea. This makes the eye very sore and may even cause an ulcer to form (see page 48).

Both conditions are treated by the doctor:

1. With antibiotic eyedrops or ointment to prevent infection.
2. Entropion can be prevented by a strip of sticky tape being attached to the lid margin and down on to the cheek; this is an excellent measure to be used until you can see a specialist.
3. If you have ectropion, you should be careful when wiping away tears. It is better to dab the closed eye rather than wipe it downwards as this tends to pull the slack lid even farther away from the eye.
4. Both conditions usually need a small surgical correction which can be carried out under a local anaesthetic.

Mistaken cases of entropion   A baby with full cheeks may appear to have the lower lids turned inwards, but this is not a case of entropion and no cause for worry. As the baby grows and the chubbiness disappears the eyelids will appear quite normal.

A further condition causing your eye to look red is acute glaucoma; but as this is an uncommon problem I shall describe it in Chapter 8, where I talk about all types of glaucoma. First I shall describe the more common disorders relating especially to children and young adults.

7 CHILDREN'S EYE PROBLEMS

Your children's health is a prime concern, and from their birth you will be concerned that they should have good sight. It is difficult for parents to assess their babies' eyesight, however, because young babies' level of vision changes rapidly over the early years.

At birth babies are able to fix their gaze on an object but it is not until they are two to three months old that they can follow a moving object with both eyes. Although they move their eyes inwards as interesting toys are brought towards them, they cannot coordinate the movement with the necessáry focusing until they are two to three years old.

In the first year of life a baby probably can only see the equivalent to the top letter on a distance vision testing chart, 6/60 (see Chapter 3). By the age of two the level has improved considerably and the child can see objects the same size as the fifth line, 6/12. It is not until the age of five that normal vision is achieved.

Testing your child's eyes

Children born in hospital have their eyes examined at birth to check for any serious abnormality. After that, there is no need to have your children's eyes tested until between the ages of three and five, when normal vision develops (except for a squint, see page 58). Children's eyes are usually tested at school clinics as early as possible. However, these are not often very thorough tests and if you are concerned that your child can't see properly you should consult your doctor as well.

Children may suffer from any of the three focusing errors, myopia, long sight or astigmatism, which I describe in Chapter 5, and may need glasses. If your child complains that he or she is having difficulty seeing, say, the blackboard at school, do make sure that this is not just attention-seeking. If there does seem to be a genuine problem, even if it is psychologically based, your doctor or eye specialist will know best how to deal with it.

Preparing for the test
If your child is only between two and five and needs a test, either for a squint or the other focusing errors, the optician or optometrist will have to take special measures. Small children tend to move their eyes around and will seldom look at one point for long. As they look around they also

alter their focus so that testing becomes impossible. To overcome this problem, eyedrops or ointment are given to dilate the pupils and stop the focusing muscle moving. This allows the specialist to assess the eyes without relying on the child's account of what he or she is seeing, which may be inaccurate – or even untrue! The temporary paralysis of the focusing muscle prevents the eye changing focus and the large pupil means the retina can be examined.

Eyedrops may be used at the first visit, or you may be given ointment to put into the eyes for several days before the test (see opposite). If you have been asked to use an ointment, remember not to put any into the eyes on the day of the test as it tends to glue the lids together and make the test more difficult to carry out.

When a child is given eyedrops or ointment the near vision becomes very blurred. This may last for twenty-four hours with some eyedrops; with others it can continue for up to a week. The longer-lasting drugs tend to be used on the first visit as they give more accurate results, while the shorter-acting ones are sometimes needed at later checks. Because of the blurring of vision it is best to arrange your visits to a specialist at times when there is no interruption in school work.

Assessing your child's vision
If your child needs glasses around the age of three they will be ordered from the results of this test. As by the age of four most children can begin to recognize the shape of letters they can take a more active part in the test, though their responses are not relied on alone (see above).

There are several ways to assess a young child's vision. In the simplest, the E test, the child is asked to hold up a cut-out E shape in the same direction as one held by the specialist. In the Sheridan Gardiner test the specialist holds up a card with letters of different sizes and asks the child to point to the same letters on a card he or she is holding.

Common eye problems in children

The red eye problems I described in Chapter 6, particularly styes, chalazion and conjuctivitis (see pages 46, 51–2) are very common in children of all ages, and I describe there how they occur and may be avoided or treated.

Apart from the focusing problems described above, there are only two common ailments that particularly affect children – squints and watering eyes. Congenital cataract and glaucoma can also occur in children but they are rare. I deal with them in Chapters 8 and 9.

Watering eyes
This is most common in young babies, usually starting soon after birth. It is due to incomplete development of the tear passages into the nose and

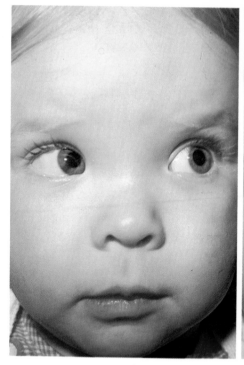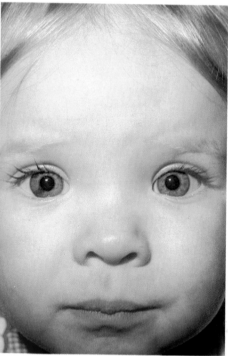

Some children seem to have a squint when they turn their eyes right or left, but their eyes are straight when they look ahead.

can affect one or both sides. The trouble often settles during the first year, but the tears may become infected, especially with a head cold. Then a sticky discharge prevents the eyes from opening.

Treatment You should take your child to the family doctor who will prescribe antibiotic eyedrops or an ointment.

It is easier if two people apply the eyedrops or ointment but it is quite possible to do it on your own. If there are two of you the method is:

1. Wrap the baby in a blanket so that the arms are firmly held;
2. Lay the baby back on the lap of the helper, who steadies the baby's head.
3. The ointment or eyedrops can then be given by the method used for adults (see page 30–1).
4. It will help if you can massage the tear sac by pressing between the side of the nose and the inner ends of the eyelids with the tip of your finger.

If you are on your own, you must wrap your baby firmly (as in 1) and rest your forearms on the blanket. This will steady your hands and prevent your baby from wriggling out of the blanket. With a small baby it is possible to hold the head between your hands while using your thumbs and first fingers to open the lids and administer the treatment.

How long should you continue treatment?   If your baby's eyes continue to be watery and sticky after about three months of treatment, the specialist may need to syringe the ducts. This will be done under a general anaesthetic and may need to be repeated several times.

Does the condition affect older children?   It is uncommon in older children unless the blockage has been allowed to continue from birth, so that later the child's tear sac may become infected.

Treating older children   The same treatment for watery eyes applies to older children. You may need to give your child eyedrops for other conditions too, such as conjunctivitis.

If you are putting drops that sting into your child's eye, say that they may sting *after* you have instilled the drops. If you mention it before using them the child is likely to screw up his or her eyes – or refuse to come near you at all!

Squints

If you have a squint, one eye looks at an object while your squinting eye points elsewhere. You may have heard other terms to describe a squint, for example strabismus, cast, turn, wall-eye or cross-eye. Some people also use the word when they mean that the eyes are screwed up against bright light, with the eyelids only half open.

A squint may be convergent, with one eye turned inwards, divergent, with one eye turned outwards, or vertical, when one eye appears higher than the other.

How common are squints?
A squint is by far the most common eye complaint in children that needs an operation. Eighty per cent of children visiting my clinic are being treated for squints.

Of the three types the convergent squint is the most common, usually occurring in children under the age of ten. I see at least twenty times as many convergent as divergent squints in children of this age. A divergent squint is most often seen in teenage children or adults; the vertical squint is rarely found in children.

When do squints occur?
Squints can occur at any age in childhood. They may be present at birth,

especially if there is a weakness of the eye muscles. This may happen if the birth has been difficult or if the delivery was by forceps.

Most often a squint is first noticed either when your child starts to focus on close objects between the age of two and three or when he or she goes to school.

Why should you suspect your child has a squint?

1. You or someone in your family may notice your child's eyes are not both pointing in the same direction. This is often more marked when your child is tired or after an illness.
2. Members of your family have had squints or had to wear glasses. Squints very often run in families.
3. Your child blinks a lot or moves his or her head from side to side to blot out double vision.
4. In an older child, perhaps in the early teens, you may get complaints of eye strain or double vision.

When is a squint not a squint?   Babies with a wide nose bridge and folds of skin which extend from the upper to the lower eyelids beside the nose often appear to have a squint. This is called epicanthus (see page 57). The eyes appear quite straight when looking to the front but on looking to the left the right eye seems to turn in more than the left eye turns out. When the child looks in the opposite direction, the left eye appears to have moved more than the right eye.

No treatment is needed as this apparent uneven movement of the eyes gradually disappears with the normal growth of the face. The idea of a 'self-righting' squint probably arose from this condition. A real squint cannot improve on its own and so if your child has epicanthus you should see a specialist to make sure that there is no underlying genuine squint.

What causes a squint?

There are many causes of squint – among them a muscle defect, congenital cataract (see Chapter 9) and meningitis, but by far the commonest is the type associated with long sight.

At birth your eye is only three-quarters the size that it will become when you are fully grown. Your eye is therefore long-sighted and to see something near you must refocus (see the diagram on page 34). There is normally a close link between the amount of focusing needed to see a near object and the angle to which the eyes must converge. If a special effort has to be made to focus on a near object because of very long sight the brain responds by too great a convergence of the eyes. The result is a convergent squint, with one eye turning inwards more than it should.

There may also be some imbalance between the muscles that move the

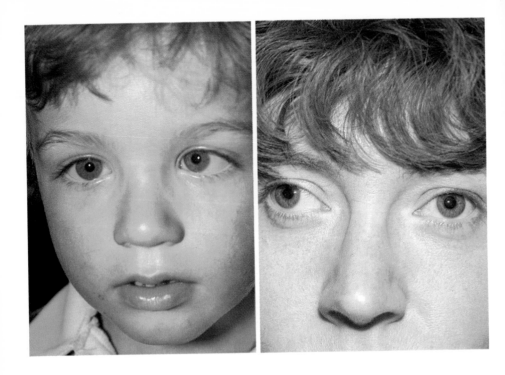

Left, a convergent squint, with the left eye turned inwards, and *right*, a divergent squint, with the left eye turned outwards.

eyes from side to side. If the muscles that turn the eyes outwards are weak there is a tendency to a convergent squint. The opposite effect occurs with weak muscles that move the eyes inwards, when a divergent squint may develop.

How does a squint affect your child's vision?

If a child has a squint the brain ignores the image from the squinting eye. This is necessary to overcome the double vision that the child begins to see as the images from both eyes are transmitted to the brain. The effect is the same as if you were looking down a microscope or sighting a rifle. You concentrate on the image from the eye that you are using even though the other eye is open and still seeing. With a squint this disregard by the brain over many months may result in a lazy eye, which is called amblyopia. If it is not treated before the age of eight the lazy eye will remain permanently weaker and nothing can ever be done to improve the level of vision.

When should you take your child for treatment?

Generally speaking the younger the child the more rapid is the development of the lazy eye. It is also true that the younger the child the easier it is to correct a lazy eye. So you should take your child to your doctor as soon as you suspect a squint.

When you take your child to the doctor and are first describing the squint, do indicate the correct eye. Remember that as you look at someone's face the right eye as you see it is in fact the left eye. This obvious fact is often overlooked by parents when it comes to describing a squint and the wrong eye is blamed.

What tests are done?

Your doctor will send you to a specialist who will usually decide at the first visit if your child has a squint. If the squint is only seen occasionally, though, it may take several visits to be sure of this.

You will also see an orthoptist who has specialized in the management of squints, and is used to dealing with children. There are various methods of testing the sight in each eye and of measuring the degree of the squint. Children usually enjoy the tests and once they have got to know the orthoptist do not mind their visits to hospital. The alignment tests sometimes take the form of looking into an instrument at a divided picture, half being visible to each eye.

It is usually helpful for a parent to accompany a baby or small child but many children behave and perform better when they are alone. Therefore do not insist on being present all the time.

Treatment

Glasses If a squint is found, the first step is to see if glasses are needed; no child is too young for the test (see page 55). If glasses are prescribed you should make certain that they are worn all the time. It may be possible later to reduce the length of time or to use them only for close work. Glasses with lenses that are very strong at the start can sometimes be weakened as the treatment proceeds.

Some convergent squints due to long sight will be cured by glasses. For those who still squint, even when wearing glasses, exercises may help but eventually an operation will be needed.

Wearing a patch If the tests show that the sight in one eye is poor, a patch is put over your child's good eye, to make the poorer one work harder. It will have to be worn for varying lengths of time each day at home. The orthoptist will show you how to cover the eye, and explain when this is to be done. Your child will be given pastimes such as tracing or writing to draw attention away from the patch and help use the other eye.

Patching may be needed for anything from six months to two years. The aim of the treatment is to bring the level of vision in the lazy or squinting eye up to that of the good eye.

Operation This will be needed if glasses and exercises have failed to control a squint. The aim of the operation is to straighten the eyes, and this is done by altering the position of the muscles that move them. It is usually performed on the squinting eye. It does not affect the sight in either eye.

In my experience two-thirds of children with squints do need an operation. Of them, two-thirds need only one operation, while the remaining third may need further surgery. This may be performed on the other eye if the maximum alteration has already been carried out on the first eye.

The operation is done under a general anaesthetic. In some hospitals you will be admitted only for the day of the operation, and be sent home when your child has recovered from the anaesthetic. In other centres you may be admitted for one or two nights.

The operated eye may be padded. It will tend to be rather red and sore and this may last for up to a month, but there won't be any real pain.

After the operation

1. If your child already has glasses make sure they are worn.
2. Give the eyedrops and/or ointment prescribed for as long as the doctor specifies.
3. Get your child back to school after a week.
4. Allow any gentle recreation and watching television.
5. Do not allow vigorous or possibly harmful sports such as football, tennis or cricket, or any swimming, while your child's eyes look red.
6. If the redness persists for as long as six weeks, even though you are using the eyedrops prescribed, and there seems to be a slight swelling, do consult your doctor.

The ideal and most usual end result of squint treatment achieves equal vision in both eyes, with the images from both joined by the brain to produce stereoscopic vision (see Chapter 1). Occasionally the brain and the eye muscles do not coordinate, even though the positioning has been put right and then we have to settle for an acceptable cosmetic appearance.

I have in these first chapters talked about problems that affect people's eyes at any time in their lives from birth to middle age – conditions that are often easily diagnosed and easily put right. I shall now describe the eye diseases which, though not unknown in younger people, are usually found in middle to old age.

8 GLAUCOMA

This is a condition with various forms, the first common in middle-aged and older people, and I shall describe this type in detail. Any variation in symptoms and treatment in the other types I describe separately, especially acute glaucoma which differs considerably from the others. The different types of glaucoma are:

1. Chronic
2. Acute
3. Secondary
4. Childhood.

Chronic glaucoma

This – also called open-angle or chronic simple glaucoma – is a slow, insidious disease which can seriously affect your sight unless it is treated. The sooner it is detected the better. This is not a condition that can finally be cured, but treatment will slow or halt its progress and ensure that your vision is not damaged.

Glaucoma affects both eyes but often one eye develops the disease before the other. It is caused by a slow rise in the pressure of the aqueous fluid within the eye due to its inability to escape through the normal drainage channels. The reason for this is unknown. In the normal healthy eye there is a balance between the rate of fluid produced in the eye and the rate at which it drains out of the eye.

How does the pressure affect the eye?
The pressure inside your eye is measured in millimetres of mercury (mm Hg). These are the same units of measurement that your doctor uses to record the blood pressure. The normal pressure level in your eye is 15 to 20 mm Hg. This can be slightly higher or lower without meaning that there is anything wrong, in the same way that some normally healthy people can be very tall or very short. In glaucoma the pressure may be up to twice the normal level.

The nutrition to the optic nerve and retina is supplied by blood pumped to your eye by the normal blood pressure. If the eye pressure is too high it is more difficult for the blood to enter, in the same way as it becomes

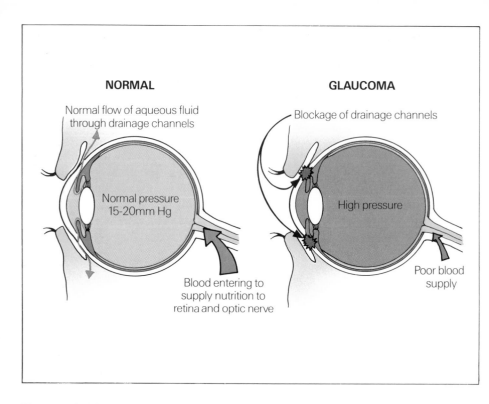

Glaucoma builds up pressure in the eye as the drainage channels become blocked.

harder to inflate a tyre when the pressure in it is already high.

As a result your optic nerve becomes starved of blood and parts of it begin to die.

Who is most at risk?
Chronic glaucoma affects about 1 per cent of the population over the age of forty. Under forty it is rare.

There is a strong tendency for the disease to run in families, so that members of a family with a glaucoma sufferer are ten times more likely to get it. This means that if you are found to have glaucoma you should make certain that your brothers, sisters and your children are examined by a specialist. Any of them under the age of forty should be examined every five years and those over forty should be seen every two years.

Chronic glaucoma is three times more common in anyone with diabetes.

What are the symptoms?
The problem with chronic glaucoma is that you may have no early symptoms; or you may only occasionally feel a slight eye ache or headache. There is even a very unusual form of the disease known as low-tension glaucoma when the pressure does not rise; but in every other respect this

64

is identical to chronic glaucoma and once diagnosed it is treated in the same way.

The loss of vision in glaucoma is slow, taking several months or even a year before it becomes really noticeable. Since it is the side vision which is affected, you are able to read normally and you are likely to be unaware of the gradual loss of vision.

Glaucoma is most often diagnosed when you attend for a sight test. The specialist may suspect the early changes of glaucoma when examining the inside of your eyes. He can confirm that you have glaucoma by measuring your eye pressure, testing your fields of vision and examining the back of your eyes.

Loss of fields of vision

If you have the early stages of the condition there may be small areas of loss of vision similar to your normal blind spot (see Chapter 3). These tend to lie above and below the central portion of your vision. If they occur in only one eye, the other eye compensates for the loss because the fields of vision of each eye overlap. But if both eyes are involved you may become aware of the blind area.

Usually you will not realize how much of your vision is missing unless it is tested by a specialist. Although you can try the tests I describe in Chapter 3, you cannot assess your own fields of vision accurately enough to be able to decide if you have glaucoma.

Testing your eye pressure

There are several methods used; the most accurate involves touching the clear window or cornea very lightly. This may sound unpleasant, but in fact it is a painless procedure. First, anaesthetic eyedrops are put into your eyes. These may sting for a few seconds but are no worse than getting soap into your eyes.

You should not be worried if you blink as the instrument used to test your eye pressure touches your cornea. The specialist can gently hold your eyelids open for the few seconds that it takes to do the test.

Another popular method involves an instrument which does not touch the eye but instead puffs a small jet of air at the cornea. This technique does not require a local anaesthetic but unfortunately it gives less accurate measurements. Most people who have experienced both methods prefer the first even though eyedrops have to be given.

Treatment

The aim of treatment is to lower the eye pressure throughout the day to a level that is no longer dangerous. This will prevent you losing more of your field of vision.

There is a normal fluctuation throughout twenty-four hours, with the pressure usually at its highest between 6 and 8 am. For this reason it is sometimes necessary to be admitted to hospital so that your eye pressure can be measured at regular intervals throughout the day.

Treatment is either with eyedrops and pills or by operation. Most eye surgeons prefer to start with medical treatment of eyedrops and pills and only recommend surgery if these fail. However, some surgeons may suggest an operation at an early stage.

Medical treatment

The eyedrops that you are given will probably be one or more of the following:

1. Pilocarpine
2. Adrenaline
3. Guanethidine
4. Timolol.

As long as the medical treatment works for you, you will have to use one of these drugs. As I said on page 63, it is not possible to have a once and for all cure, but treatment prevents your vision from getting worse.

The pills that are given will be one of the following:

1. Acetazolamide
2. Dichlorphenamide.

Each has its role in treating glaucoma and both have their side-effects. If you get side-effects, tell your doctor and he or she will change the treatment to one better suited to you.

Eyedrops

For instructions on applying eyedrops and ointment, see Chapter 4.

Pilocarpine This is the most commonly prescribed drug and is made up in strengths of ½ to 6 per cent. The strength you are given will depend on your particular need. The drops last for six hours only and therefore should be taken every six hours. In practice, of course, this is not possible as most people sleep longer than six hours. Here is a satisfactory compromise:

Dose 1: 6 to 7 am
Dose 2: 12 to 1 midday
Dose 3: 5 to 6 pm
Dose 4: 11 pm or immediately before going to bed.

It is not known how pilocarpine lowers the eye pressure but it acts on the muscle surrounding the lens and the effect is constriction of your pupil and alteration of the focus of your eye.

Constriction of your pupil reduces the light entering your eyes and dims your vision. This dimming lasts for up to two hours after the eyedrops have been instilled and causes most difficulty after dark. You may also notice colours become less intense. The effect on your vision will be worse if you also suffer from cataract (opacity in your lens – see Chapter 9).

Alteration of the focus of your eye is uncommon after the age of fifty-five, but it may be a drawback if you develop glaucoma in your forties when alteration in the focus makes you shortsighted. Distant objects become blurred for up to two hours and this may restrict activities such as driving.

Side-effects   Some people get a slight ache in their eyes using pilocarpine due to constriction of the muscles inside the eye. Sometimes the pain may be more severe although this is rare. Usually any slight discomfort wears off after a week or ten days' treatment.

Adrenaline   This drug is often given in addition to pilocarpine and works by decreasing the amount of fluid produced in the eye and increasing its draining away. It dilates the pupil. The eyedrops, of ½ to 2 per cent strength, are used every twelve hours. If you are prescribed adrenaline make sure that:

1. The container is kept tightly sealed, cool and dark. A refrigerator is a good place.
2. If the solution changes to an amber colour you should replace it as the drug will have become inactive.
3. If you also have to take pilocarpine put the adrenaline in ten to fifteen minutes after using the pilocarpine.

Side-effects   Adrenaline tends to sting when used and can make your eyes rather red and gritty. You may also get slight eye ache and brow ache. Occasionally palpitations, trembling and perspiration occur, and when it is used for long periods small black deposits develop inside the lower lids. These are noticeable but are no cause for alarm, as they are only due to a chemical change in the drug which causes a deposit of black pigment.

Guanethidine   This drug is less often used than the first two, but when taken with adrenaline it can enhance the action. The eyedrops are supplied combined with adrenaline in strengths of 1 to 5 per cent and are used twice each day.

Side-effects   These are the same as with adrenaline. Some people also notice slight drooping of the upper eyelids. It does not affect your vision and lasts only as long as you are taking the drug.

Timolol This most recent addition to the anti-glaucoma drugs belongs to a group known as beta blockers and has provided glaucoma sufferers with good eye pressure control without the unpleasant side-effects of the other eyedrops.

Timolol eyedrops are either a ¼ or ½ per cent strength and need only be used twice a day. The control of the pressure is more successful than with twice-a-day adrenaline. Your pupils do not constrict and you do not get the same blurring as with pilocarpine.

Side-effects Timolol can affect people who have heart trouble or breathing difficulties so it cannot be taken by them. There are other reported problems such as discomfort in the eyes and general lethargy but these seem to be rare.

Which eyedrops?
Your doctor will prescribe the best for your particular condition.

The advantages of pilocarpine are that it is a very effective drug and has less effect on your general health than the others, so it is best for older people with glaucoma.

Adrenaline and guanethidine are excellent alternatives for people who find the four-times-a-day treatment of pilocarpine difficult to remember, but who cannot take timolol because of its side-effects.

Timolol is the ideal drug for young people with glaucoma who find the dimming and blurring of pilocarpine unacceptable. But the cost of the drug is high and this makes some doctors reluctant to prescribe it.

Pills
Both acetazolamide and dichlorphenamide lower the eye pressure by reducing the amount of fluid produced in your eyes. They are used as additional treatment to eyedrops. The pills act for about six hours so that you may have to take up to four each day.

Acetazolamide is also made in a capsule form which delays the release of the drug so that twice daily treatment is possible.

Side-effects The most marked and common side-effect is tingling in the hands, feet and face. This is usually tolerable but occasionally may become unpleasant enough for you to have to stop the treatment. Indigestion, loss of appetite and weight loss are less common than the tingling sensation.

Both drugs act on the kidneys, increasing salt and water loss in the urine so that you may notice that you have to pass water more frequently. Potassium is also lost like salt and may need to be replaced if you are on the drugs for a long time. This can be done by taking potassium as a medicine or more naturally in your diet. Bananas and oranges are particularly rich in potassium and pleasanter than swallowing a pill.

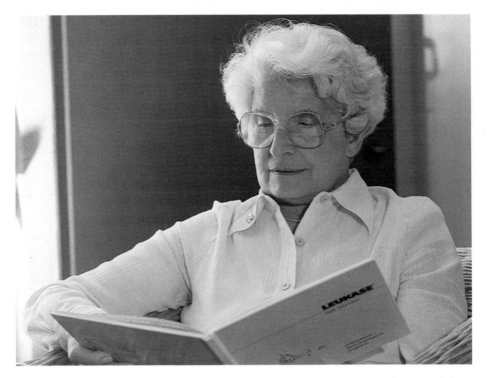

For the first few weeks after an eye operation you should relax as much as possible.

Surgical treatment of glaucoma: when should it be given?

A few eye surgeons suggest surgical treatment when glaucoma is first diagnosed without even trying to control the pressure with eyedrops. The majority recommend an operation when they feel that the eye pressure is no longer controlled by eyedrops and pills. This failure of medical treatment may be because:

1. The pressure remains too high and your vision is getting worse even when you are taking the maximum dose of drugs.
2. You have unpleasant side-effects from the drugs.
3. The specialist feels that you may not be able to keep to his instructions owing to physical causes, such as arthritis, making the instillation of eyedrops difficult; or to forgetfulness so that you do not take the drugs regularly.

When eyedrops are no longer effective, treatment by laser and eyedrops is often successful and avoids the need for surgery. This is done under local anaesthetic. The aim of surgical treatment is the same as with medical treatment – to lower the eye pressure to a level that is no longer dangerous.

About two-thirds of operations for glaucoma control the pressure, most of the remaining third will be controlled with additional eyedrops and less than 10 per cent need a further operation; and this is usually successful.

There are several types of operation, and all reduce the pressure by creating a new way for the fluid to escape from your eye.

The most popular method is trabeculectomy, as it lowers the pressure with the minimum of accompanying problems and the highest chance of success. The operation lasts about half an hour and is usually performed under general anaesthetic. If your health is poor it is possible to carry out successful and painless surgery under a local anaesthetic.

After the operation   Your eye will be padded all the time for two to three days and at night for a fortnight. You will stay in hospital for about a week.

It is inevitable that your vision will change after the operation. As your eye heals it changes shape and so the focus alters. This means that you may require a change of lenses after about two months, when the healing is complete.

You will be given eyedrops to help the soreness and inflammation after the operation and these should be effective within a few weeks. Do report any stickiness or suspected conjunctivitis as your eyes will be susceptible to infection.

You will be able to return to work within a month, but be sensible and do not strain yourself or put yourself under great pressure. The advice I give for people who have had a cataract operation (see Chapter 9) applies as much here.

How you can help in the long term

1. Continue to use your eyedrops regularly. If you miss an occasional eyedrop it will not matter but if you let this happen repeatedly your eye pressure will rise and you will slowly lose your sight.
2. Do not drink large volumes of fluid in a short space of time as this may raise your eye pressure. Not more than 1 pt (500 cc) of fluid may be safely taken over a quarter of an hour.
3. Normal everyday activities, even strenuous ones, and activities involving close work such as reading are quite safe, but you shouldn't overdo things. The exercises described by Jane Madders in *Stress and Relaxation*, in this series, will help you relax.

Other types of glaucoma: acute glaucoma

Also called narrow-angle or congestive glaucoma, this gives you an extremely painful red eye with your vision reduced so that you can barely see light, but unlike chronic glaucoma it can be cured.

It happens suddenly, when the fluid inside your eye cannot drain away. The pupil dilates and the iris blocks the normal drainage channels. This is more likely to happen in the short eye of someone who has long sight (see Chapter 5). It can affect one or both eyes.

The first sign is the appearance of haloes of coloured light like rainbows around lights during the evening. People say that when they have been watching an exciting movie in a darkened room, tending to make the pupils dilate, they get this effect. The eye may also ache slightly. The symptoms usually settle overnight as your pupils constrict during sleep. These mild episodes can happen over several months before you have an acute attack.

The acute attack develops over several hours with such severe pain that it may make you vomit. In fact, some people are so ill that the eye can be overlooked as the cause of the troubles.

Who gets acute glaucoma?   It is a very uncommon condition compared to chronic glaucoma. There is only one case of acute glaucoma for every four or five of chronic glaucoma. About 0.5 per cent of the entire population may get it. It usually occurs in middle-aged, long-sighted people, and for no known reason is more common in women. It does not run in families.

Immediate action is needed to save the sight. Your doctor will arrange to have you admitted to hospital for intensive treatment with eyedrops. You will also be given an injection to help to lower the pressure and another to help the pain and nausea.

Eventually, when the acute stage is over, you will need an operation. This will both cure the acute condition and prevent a recurrence. The operation can be carried out under a general or local anaesthetic. A small piece of iris is removed from your affected eye. It will be necessary to treat the other eye in the same way, as that will also be at risk.

Recent developments have made it possible to burn a small hole in the iris with a laser beam, rather like burning a leaf by concentrating the rays of the sun with a magnifying glass. This has the same effect as removing a piece by operation and can be performed under local anaesthetic. It may one day replace the conventional procedure.

You stay in hospital for only three or four days for the operation. Afterwards you will need to use ointment or eyedrops for a few weeks, and should take life gently until any soreness has gone (see page 69).

Secondary glaucoma

This occurs when the eye's fluid pressure rises as a result of another eye condition. The cause is usually blockage in the drainage mechanism. This may follow a blow to your eye causing bleeding inside the front half of your eye when red blood cells tend to clog the drainage channels.

Inflammation inside your eye (see Iritis, Chapter 5), can produce the same effect due to blockage by white blood cells.

The condition will be diagnosed when you are having your eye examined for the other problem; eye pressure tests are made as a matter of course when you have a red eye or iritis. You will be given eyedrops and ointment, as for chronic glaucoma, to treat secondary glaucoma.

Childhood glaucoma

Glaucoma can also occur in children but is fortunately very uncommon; I have only seen one case in the last ten years. It tends to affect boys more than girls (although we don't know why this is so) and may occur in one or both eyes. It is due to faulty development of the eye, so that the aqueous fluid is unable to drain away. As the pressure rises the eye enlarges and the clear cornea becomes cloudy. This increase in size gives the condition the name 'ox eye'. The child dislikes bright light and tends to screw up his or her eyes even in normal daylight.

These symptoms will be obvious to parents and are almost certain to be due to glaucoma. An immediate appointment should be arranged with your family doctor or with your eye specialist.

Early treatment by operation is essential if the sight is to be saved. This can be performed even in the first few weeks after birth.

Although, as we have seen, all conditions of glaucoma can't be cured, something can be done to prevent your eyes being seriously damaged, and provided you follow the treatment prescribed for you properly, you should maintain a reasonable level of eyesight for a good length of time. The conditions I describe in the next chapter, cataract and macular degeneration, are even more common in older people than glaucoma. But cataract can be reversed with more effective and, for the person concerned, more exciting results.

9 CATARACT AND MACULAR DEGENERATION

Nearly everyone has heard the word cataract. Many people link cataract with operation – yet this is only done for a minority of people with it.

What is a cataract?
A cataract is a cloudiness or opacity in the lens of your eye (see diagram on page 11). It is caused by a change of the lens protein which becomes opaque, similar to the way the white of an egg changes from clear to white when cooked.

Who gets it?
If you are born with a cataract it is called congenital. This type is most

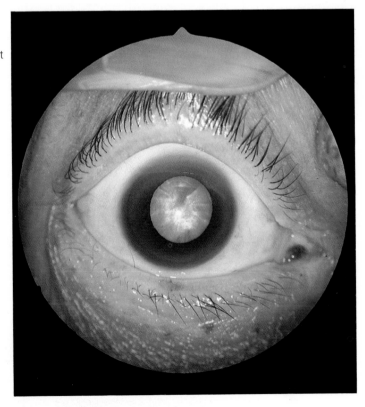

The black pupil has turned white due to the development of a cataract.

commonly seen as a result of maternal German measles during pregnancy, which fortunately is rare due to widespread vaccination. The extent of a congenital cataract may vary from a small opacity which has little or no effect on your vision to complete whiteness of the lens which severely affects the sight and requires an operation.

Cataracts that develop in childhood are rare, but in adults they become more common with increasing age. Between the ages of fifty and sixty about 65 per cent of both men and women have some cataract and this rises to 95 per cent over the age of sixty-five.

Having a cataract does not mean inevitable loss of sight or impending operation. Admittedly, if you are over sixty, you may experience a change in vision which eventually can be helped by removal of the cataract, but for most people a cataract may at the worst cause some difficulty in seeing, and for many it goes completely unnoticed.

How will a cataract affect your vision?

The change in your sight will depend on the position of the cataract. One on the central line of vision will cause more difficulties than one at the edge of your lens – rather like a scratch in the centre of a glasses' lens causes more trouble than one to the side, which may not be noticed. The following effects can occur together or singly if you have a cataract, though the first, blurring, you will always experience.

In the early stages you may notice only slight blurring of your vision. There may also be some dimming of colours which may take on a brownish hue like the later paintings of the early nineteenth-century English landscape artist, J.M.W. Turner. As the cataract increases, the haziness slowly becomes worse and the level of lighting becomes critical, so that too little light makes seeing difficult while too much causes dazzle. These effects of light make night driving dangerous. You may also start to notice either haloes or a bright star-like appearance with oncoming headlights or around street lamps.

Certain types of cataract cause double vision so that you see two faces where there is only one on the television screen or a ghosting around the edge of an object. This occurs when the cataract is in the centre of the lens like a flaw in a gemstone.

One type of cataract causes hardening of the centre of your lens, and this is called nuclear sclerosis. It alters the focus of the eye so that you become short-sighted. You may then find that where you previously needed reading glasses you can manage better without them – some compensation for the development of the cataract!

When the whole of your lens becomes cloudy, it is impossible to see any detail and you may only be aware of a light in front of you. This is of course one extreme and between it and normal vision there are all gradations of haziness. You may be able to live with the haziness you have, depending on your particular visual needs.

How quickly does it develop? A cataract can take anything from a few months to thirty years to develop.

Learning to live with your cataract

Because the majority are never dense enough to make an operation necessary most people have to learn to live with their cataracts. The following points will help you to make the most of your sight if you have a cataract that does not need an operation.

1. Your eyes work by light – too little and you can't see, too much and they become dazzled. This applies to everyone but particularly to people with a cataract. Get your lighting right – it is the single most important point for coping with your cataract.
2. Out of doors avoid light shining directly on your eyes. This is particularly troublesome when the sun is low in the sky in spring and autumn. You will probably see better on an overcast cloudy day than in bright sunshine.
3. Wear a hat with a brim, a tennis eye-shield or a baseball cap with a peak. If you don't want to use one of these, you may improve your vision simply by shielding your eyes with your hand.
4. When driving use the sun visor if the light is at all bright and not just when the sun is shining.
5. Sunglasses or tinted lenses may help to reduce dazzle when you are outside, but indoors you will usually see better with clear lenses. The choice of how dark your lenses should be is a personal one. Ask your optician or optometrist to show you the range available. Photochromic lenses that change depending on the brightness of the light may also help (see Chapter 5).
6. Indoors it is easier to arrange your lighting so that your eyes are protected from direct light. You will often find that shaded lights are better than unshaded ones.
7. When you are watching television do not have any light in front of you. You need only the light from the television set.
8. When reading you must have the light shining over your shoulders on to the book, with your face shaded. Trying to read with only a bright ceiling light may be difficult. An adjustable reading lamp is best as you can position it near enough to the print. The distance from lamp to book is critical. If you halve this distance, the amount of light on the page is quadrupled. Put another way, a 60 watt bulb at 3 ft (1 m) gives the same light as 240 watts from 6 ft (2 m). Most floor lamps have light bulbs of only 100–150 watts, which may be quite inadequate when placed 6 to 8 ft away (2 to 2.5 m).
9. Your reading may be helped by reducing the glare from the paper, particularly when it is shiny. Cover half the page with a piece of matt black card or even cut a slit 1 × 6 in (2 × 15 cm) through which to

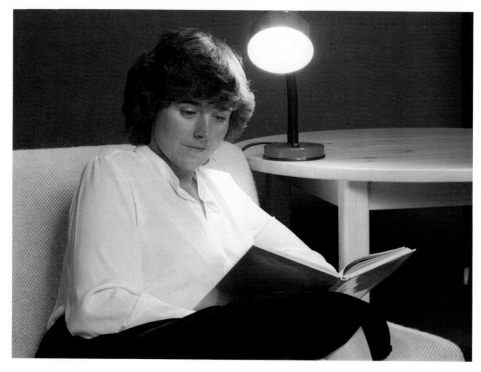

If you have a cataract, correct positioning of your reading light is essential.

view the print. This will prevent reflection of unwanted light from the remainder of the page from striking your eyes.

10. Do not panic if you think that your vision has suddenly become worse. It is almost invariably due to a change in lighting. Artificial lighting is usually less effective than natural daylight, so your sight may seem worse when you go indoors. Make the most of natural light by drawing curtains well back and not using net curtains.

Treatment
The only effective treatment for a dense cataract is removal by an operation. Although there have been claims that cataract can be prevented and cleared with drugs and eyedrops, these are quack remedies that should definitely be avoided.

When to operate
The popular idea that you must wait until your cataract is 'ripe' is wrong. The correct time for operation is when you are no longer able to see to continue with everyday living.

In every case of cataract, the specialist is balancing the advantages of

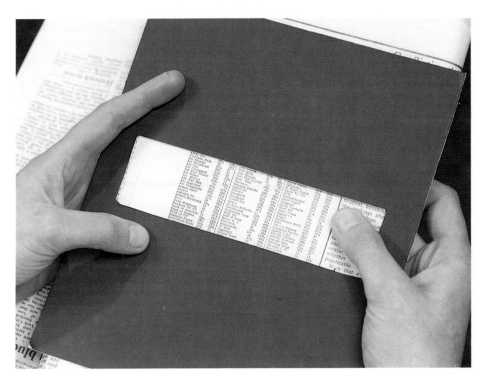

A piece of black card placed over a shiny page helps reduce the glare.

better vision after surgery against the risks that accompany even the simplest operations. In general the younger you are the more benefit you are likely to get.

What the operation entails

Cataract surgery involves removing the cloudy lens from your eye and replacing it with glasses, a contact lens or a plastic lens within your eye; a cataract is not merely a skin that can be scraped or peeled away.

The operation can be performed under a local or general anaesthetic. Many people feel that under local anaesthetic they will be unable to keep their eyes open or that they may move around too much. However the local anaesthetic will prevent any movement of your eye and will allow the surgeon to hold open your eyelids to operate without you feeling any pain.

There are several types of operation. Each one takes about half an hour and each involves a different length of stay in hospital.

1. The most commonly performed operation involves removing the entire lens and this means that a large opening must be made. You will probably be kept in hospital for about one week following surgery.

2. If your specialist suggests that your vision is best corrected with a plastic lens in your eye you will have only part of the lens removed, leaving the outer rim. This operation will also mean a week's stay in hospital.
3. A few eye hospitals have equipment that can break up and suck out the cataract. This is called phakoemulsification, and only a small opening is needed to introduce the instrument into the eye. As a result your stay in hospital is only forty-eight hours or even less. Unfortunately, not everyone's eyes are suited to this treatment.

You have at least a 90 per cent chance of success with a cataract operation – and even if your reading vision is not entirely restored due to a retinal cause such as macular degeneration (see page 82), your general vision will be enormously improved.

After the operation

Recent advances with the operating microscope, very fine instruments and stitches have made it possible to sew up your eye so that you can get out of bed the day after your operation. You can begin to move around much sooner and more freely than used to be the case after cataract surgery.

The operated eye will be padded for four to five days. There is remarkably little discomfort to your eye and therefore there is a tendency for you to forget the eye and do too much. You should not attempt to bend down to pick up anything from the ground, and you should try to avoid coughing, sneezing and straining. During your hospital stay do not read with your other eye since the jerky movements of scanning the words are also performed by the operated eye.

In general, try to remember that although you feel well in yourself, your eye has undergone major surgery and must be given a chance to heal.

It will be necessary to use eyedrops for three to four weeks to keep your eye free from infection and lessen the redness produced by the operation. If you notice any stickiness and seem to be developing conjunctivitis, do consult your specialist.

After your discharge from hospital continue taking the same care that you took in hospital, especially for the first two weeks. After that you may gradually increase your activities, so that by six weeks you are back to a more or less normal sedentary routine. It is wise to avoid particularly strenuous activities such as sport or vigorous work for several weeks longer, but after three weeks you can certainly have your hair washed, although you should not lean far forward over the basin.

Correcting your vision after the operation

After your cataract has been removed you will be able to see shapes but no detail until you are given an alternative lens to focus the image on your retina. There are three ways this can be done and your surgeon will tell you which is most suitable for you:

1. Glasses
2. Contact lens
3. Lens implant.

Glasses

Most people who have cataract surgery wear glasses to correct their vision. Two pairs are needed – one for distance vision and another for close work – but these can be combined as bifocal lenses. The lenses are usually plastic because their thickness would make glass too heavy. The weight can be further reduced by having the thick part of the lens limited to a small central area.

Possible problems In addition to their thickness, which is unattractive, the lenses also produce certain visual problems which may make wearing them difficult.

The image that you see with cataract glasses is one-third larger than you were previously used to seeing. This makes glasses impossible to use if you have had a cataract removed from one eye while the other eye is normal, as your brain will be trying to look at an object and seeing it a different size with each eye.

Glasses give good vision when you are looking through the centre of the lens but your view of life is very different when you turn your eyes to the sides. Horizontal lines appear to curve upwards at the ends and vertical ones tend to bow to one side. This can make doorways appear alarmingly narrow from a distance but they revert to their normal shape as you approach them.

You will be given a temporary pair of glasses while still in hospital. These will give you clearer definition but do not be upset if you find that your vision is still rather blurred. As your eye heals it changes shape and alters its focus, so you have to wait six or eight weeks before you are given your permanent glasses. Everything will look much sharper when you are wearing them but even these may need a slight alteration after a further six months.

Adapting to glasses After reading about all these problems you will probably wonder how anyone manages to see with glasses after cataract surgery. Yet it is amazing how well your brain is able to adapt, even though at first you may think you will never be able to cope.

It may help if you start by wearing your distance glasses while sitting indoors, perhaps watching television. You will find one part of the lens gives you the sharpest view. When you want to look to one side, turn your head rather than your eyes so that you remain looking through the same point on the lens.

As your confidence grows, wear the glasses while moving around indoors and when you feel able, try them outside. It is sensible to have someone with you when you try to cross a road for the first time, as vehicles and pedestrians may keep appearing and disappearing in your side vision. This feeling of wearing blinkers is enough to stop some people wanting to drive, from lack of confidence. As long as you adjust to your glasses properly and feel happy about driving, there is no reason why you should not go back to it. But don't forget to tell your insurance company about your operation to make sure you remain insured if you return to driving.

Once your eye has healed you can start playing sports again – except of course the more violent ones such as football or squash. For these it will be necessary to wear contact lenses.

Contact lenses

Contact lenses overcome most of the problems that you might have with cataract glasses, but unfortunately they introduce a few new difficulties. All types of contact lenses can be used after a cataract operation – hard, soft, gas-permeable or extended-wear types may be recommended, depending on which is suitable for you (see Chapter 5).

Advantages of contact lenses

1. Since a contact lens is in nearly the same position as your eye lens, the difference in the size of the image that you see compared with normal is negligible. This means that it is quite possible to see with both eyes, after surgery to one eye, by using a contact lens for the operated eye.
2. Since the contact lens moves with your eye you always remain looking through the centre of the lens. This overcomes the distorting effects of glasses lenses and allows you to have normal all round vision.
3. It is often easier to tolerate a contact lens after a cataract operation than before, since many of the nerves that provide the feeling in your cornea are cut.

Disadvantages

1. You need to be able to insert and remove the contact lens each day, and to tolerate the lens on your eye. The handling of the lens is quickly learned but may be difficult to perform if your fingers are stiff with arthritis or if your remaining vision is poor. However, you can have a special pair of glasses with the lower half of the frame cut away on the cataract side. This allows you to see with the other eye to handle and insert the contact lens.
2. Contact lenses correct only your distance vision so that it is still neces-

sary to wear reading glasses as well as your contact lenses.
3. If you have had both eyes operated on for cataract you must have glasses to use when you have removed the contact lenses.
4. Even though you may normally wear your contact lenses all day, removing them only when you go to bed, you may be forced to manage without them if you get something in your eyes.

There is no doubt that for anyone under sixty contact lenses are the ideal method of correcting the vision after cataract surgery. They give the best possible visual results with the fewest adverse effects.

Lens implant
The idea of replacing the lens that has developed a cataract with an artificial lens inside the eye was first suggested in 1948 by the London eye surgeon, Mr Harold Ridley. The early results were discouraging but in the last ten years, with the use of improved microsurgical instruments and different lenses, this method of correcting vision after cataract surgery has become well established.

The plastic lens implant is usually inserted during the operation to remove the cataract. The new lens is fixed in your eye in approximately the same position as your own lens. It corrects the focus for your distance vision and you wear additional glasses for close work.

It is possible to fit implanted lenses to both eyes if you have cataracts in both, but personally I do not favour this because of practical difficulties (see below).

After the operation
You should take the same precautions in the first few weeks after the implant operation as I recommend after all cataract operations (see page 78). If you are given eyedrops to use, make sure that you do. Some drops will be to lessen the redness while others are sometimes needed to keep the pupil constricted so that the lens implant is held in position.

What are the advantages of a lens implant?

1. The results of an implant can be very rewarding as you are able to see as soon as your eye is uncovered after your operation.
2. There are none of the distortions produced by glasses and no need to bother with putting lenses in and taking them out, as with contact lenses.

What are the disadvantages?

1. This method is only suitable for a minority of people because it is essential to have a completely healthy eye apart from the cataract.

2. The implanted lens can act like a foreign body and cause inflammation in your eye. This may be difficult to control, even with eyedrops.
3. The lens may become displaced so that it can no longer function as a lens. If this happens the lens may rub on the inside of your eye, resulting in cloudiness of your cornea, and you will have to have another operation to remove or reposition the implanted lens.

I recommend lens implants only for people over the age of sixty-five whom I consider unsuitable for glasses or contact lenses.

Macular degeneration

The macula is the most sensitive central area of your retina that is used for direct vision like reading. Degeneration of this area happens as part of the normal ageing of the body – like grey hairs or wrinkles – mainly after the age of sixty-five. One in four people over sixty-five are affected and this increases to one in three after the age of eighty. Because it happens at this time of life it often accompanies the development of a cataract.

Symptoms
You will notice a gradual deterioration in the central vision. Straight lines seem to develop a kink and objects appear smaller, with an alteration in the normal colours. One eye is always affected earlier than the other.

These early symptoms give way to a haziness or greyness at the centre of your vision that is eventually replaced by a central blind area. The timing of these changes varies considerably, as does the final effect on your sight. It may be several years before you notice any marked change; but a sudden drop in vision may happen, which is caused by bleeding into the retina (see also page 98). Although both eyes will be affected eventually it can be ten years or longer before the sight of the second eye is involved.

Regardless of the outcome, you should remember that even though your central vision may be severely affected your side vision will remain normal. This prevents you from knocking into furniture or into people in a crowded street.

Treatment
There is no treatment that can prevent macular degeneration, but you can do a lot to make the most of whatever sight you have.

1. If one eye is badly affected it may help to shut it or cover it when you are watching television or trying to read. This prevents the central blur from interfering with the clear view from your better eye, and will throw no extra strain on it.

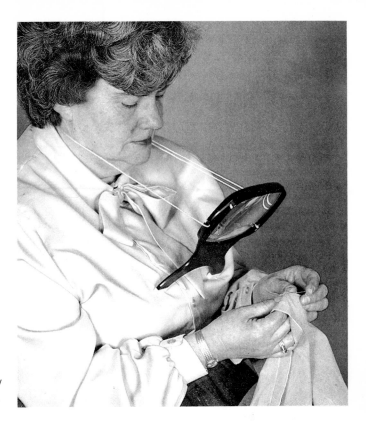

This powerful magnifier is one of the many useful low vision aids available.

2. Do not limit your reading to try to save your failing sight – your eyes are not going to wear out. Use them as normally as your level of vision permits.
3. Make sure that you have a good light placed behind your head. The advice about correct lighting for cataracts also applies to macular degeneration (see page 75).
4. Your vision may be improved with special glasses to enlarge the image. These are called low vision aids (LVAs) and can be used for near or distance vision.

Low vision aids: near vision

- The simplest is a magnifying glass. If the lens is small it can be held in your hand and kept in your pocket or handbag.
- Larger lenses can be mounted on various types of stand and some incorporate a light. They may be suspended round your neck by a cord and balanced so that you have both hands free.
- Stronger reading glasses may help, but the more powerful lenses mean that you have to hold the print much closer.

Distance vision

- LVAs for distance vision can be added to a spectacle frame so that only one eye is used. The device is a small telescope and you can adjust it for seeing in the distance or for reading or watching television by changing the lens on the front. With the enlarged image you get a restriction of the field of vision so these lenses cannot be worn for walking around.
- A telescope small enough to be carried in the hand can be used to read bus numbers or street names.
- Higher magnification – up to sixty times – can be achieved with closed-circuit television. Ordinary print is held under a televison camera and the enlarged image is shown on a television screen. This is of course a very expensive aid and is only available for people who need it especially for their work, for example, if they have to do a lot of reading.

Where to obtain LVAs

Simple LVAs such as magnifying glasses can be bought from any large stores, but the more sophisticated devices are usually supplied through eye clinics in hospitals.

Using LVAs

As with all new equipment, low vision aids require determination from the user if they are to be successful. Elderly people often lack the motivation to persevere. If your specialist has recommended an LVA for you, don't give up. Practise regularly every day and you will in the end appreciate the enormous advantage of being able to continue with many everyday activities.

10 EYE INJURIES

Although your eyes are protected from damage by the surrounding bone of your eyebrows, cheeks and nose, and against dust by your eyelashes, there are plenty of occasions when they are in danger of being injured, for example, while gardening, walking or riding in woods, or if you work with metal or glass. But the majority of serious eye injuries are avoidable provided you take proper care.

Minor injury

A common problem that everyone gets some time is a small foreign body blowing into the eye. This may be a small particle such as grit, paint, rust

How to get a foreign body out of your eye.

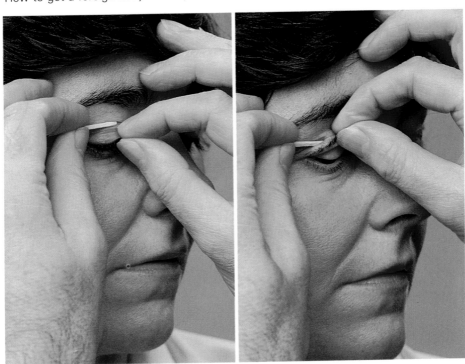

or dust, depending on what you are doing at the time. Your eye will be intensely painful, hurting with each blink, and it will water profusely.

Treatment

1. Allow your eye to water a lot, and the foreign body may be washed out by the tears; do not use an eye bath to wash your eye as this might make it even more sore (see Chapter 3).

2. Failing this, if you can see the particle on the white of your eye or your lower lid, use a clean handkerchief or tissue to coax it out.

3. If the particle is caught under the upper lid hold the lashes of your upper lid firmly and pull the lid down over the lower lid lashes. Repeat several times and you may be able to dislodge the particle.

4. If this does not succeed you must get someone to look under your upper lid by:

• Holding the eyelids of the upper lid firmly;
• Using a matchstick to press against the upper lid about half an inch (1 cm) up from the margin of the lid;
• At the same time lifting the lashes gently forwards and upwards, while you keep looking down as far as possible.

This will turn the lid over so that its inner surface can be seen. Wipe the foreign body away with a clean handkerchief or tissue. If no foreign body is visible it is still worth wiping this surface of the lid in case a particle the same colour as the lid is trapped there.

Any discomfort should settle within a few hours; but if your eye continues to be painful you should go to your doctor. If the foreign body is on the clear cornea, leave it alone and speak to your doctor or go to the casualty department in a hospital at once.

Injury to the outside of the eye

Cuts   Cuts around the outside of your eyes tend to bleed profusely but fortunately this also means that they heal very well. See your doctor if the cut is large and near the eye as the blood may hide more serious damage to your eyeball.

Injuries to the bones around your eyes   After a blow to the area around your eyes, such as from a fist, you may get double vision. This is either because the muscles moving your eyes become bruised and the eyes cannot move together or, which is less likely, the bone beneath your eye may be broken. This will trap one of the eye muscles in the crack in the bone, and will also cause you to see double, as you are unable to move your eye normally.

Fortunately both these problems clear up on their own, although occasionally people need an operation when a broken bone becomes very displaced.

Injuries from blunt objects   This may be caused by any number of circumstances. In the home, falls, chopping wood, the upturned garden rake or even carelessness in opening a bottle of champagne are possible causes, while at work there are innumerable sources of possible trouble. Vigorous sports such as tennis, squash, football and boxing account for a large number of this type of injury. Your eye may be damaged in one of several ways:

1. Bleeding from tearing of blood vessels in the coloured iris is common with blunt object injuries. This may vary in severity from a slight leakage of blood which causes mild blurring of vision to a big haemorrhage with the blood filling the space in front of the iris (called hyphaema) and causing complete loss of vision.
2. The iris may be damaged so as to produce enlargement of the pupil. This is usually permanent.
3. If the edge of the iris is torn double vision is likely.
4. Injury to your lens may cause a cataract, with gradual loss of vision.
5. If the retina is torn you may develop a retinal detachment (see page 90).

Treatment   Because of the potentially serious nature of this type of injury you should always get medical attention. Only if you have no more than minor bruising of the lids and no interference with your vision, is it safe to wait for the swelling to subside naturally.

You will need close supervision in hospital if you have extensive bleeding because of the risk of complications: another haemorrhage within the first week as a result of trying to be too active is a great danger. Rest in bed is therefore essential.

Treatment for cataract or retinal detachment will be given, as I describe in Chapter 9 and on page 91, if either of these is diagnosed.

Abrasions

This is an injury to your cornea rather like a graze on your skin – though of course there will be no bleeding from the cornea.

Abrasion can be the result of various accidents:

- a blow from a twig
- a displaced contact lens
- a baby's fingernails
- playing with a pet animal

- brushing your hair
- applying mascara to your eyelashes.

An abrasion will cause the same symptoms as a foreign body in your eye – pain and watering. Often it feels as if there is something under your upper lid, but this is because the pain occurs when the lid moves over the damaged cornea.

Treatment   If the injury is slight the abrasion will heal over within six hours. It will help and also be more comfortable if you keep your eye closed, preferably with a pad. You can make a pad of cotton wool between two layers of gauze, or failing that, use a clean handkerchief folded into a triangle and taped in a position to cover your eyeball (see illustration). The purpose of the pad is to keep your eye closed and so help the healing process.
  If the pain persists longer than six hours see your doctor.

Recurrent erosion   You may after an abrasion have later episodes of discomfort. The usual story is that your eye becomes painful suddenly at

A properly positioned pad protects an injured eye.

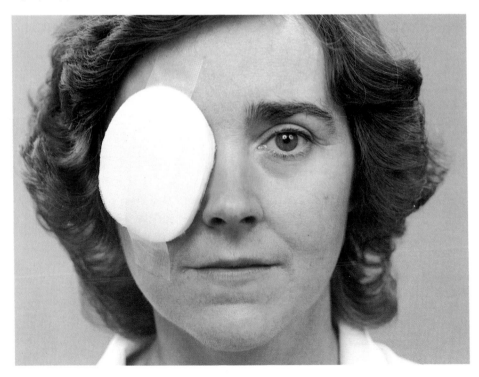

night so that it wakes you. Alternatively it may become sore and start watering as soon as you get up. These symptoms often clear completely within two to three hours, only to start again another night.

This is due to incomplete healing of an abrasion of your cornea and is called recurrent erosion. It can be treated by your doctor with antibiotic ointment. You need to apply the ointment at night for six to eight weeks.

Injuries that penetrate the eye

Injuries that penetrate any part of your eye are extremely serious and need immediate attention. These injuries are, though, far less common than damage from blunt objects: I see four to five as many blunt object as penetrating injuries. But of the people with penetrating injuries at least one in five is a child.

The danger in having an eye penetrated is not just from the damage to the structure of the eye but also because of the risk of infection getting inside the eye. In the past people's sight was frequently lost. Fortunately many eyes can now be saved due to improved surgical techniques and new antibiotics.

You might think it impossible for anyone to be unaware of being hit in the eye, but this can happen. Very small splinters of metal can enter the eye with the minimum of pain and may leave hardly a mark on the outside of the eye. Occasionally cuts in the eyelids that bleed copiously may mask far more serious damage to the eyeball.

Commonest causes

At home   There are many potential dangers: in the house, pointed knives, forks, scissors, pins, needles, sharp pencils, dangerous toys and DIY tools; in the garden, rotary lawn mowers, hedge cutters and grass trimmers with rotating nylon strands; and sticks, stones and fragments of metal or nylon that can be thrown against the eyes with sufficient force to penetrate. Here the garden débris almost invariably causes infection.

At work the commonest penetrating injuries are caused by hammers and drills. Sharp particles thrown out from the drilling can penetrate your eyes if they're not protected. The extremely high speed of the machines makes the fragments very hot, so that they are usually sterile and do not introduce infection. However, certain metals, particularly iron and copper, disintegrate if left in the eye. This will cause severe inflammation and possibly blindness.

Car injuries   The car is responsible for an ever-increasing number of eye injuries. At least one in every ten accidents results in injury to the eyes. This may vary from minor bruising to extensive penetrating injuries.

The most frequent injury is to the front-seat passenger, the head hitting the windscreen which results in horizontal cuts across the forehead and eyelids and often involves the eyeballs.

Treatment

1. Cover the injured eye with a sterile dressing, which can be bought at a pharmacy, or a clean handkerchief or pad you have made yourself (see page 88).
2. *Do not* use any eyedrops.
3. If there is bleeding it will be necessary to apply some pressure to stop it by means of a bandage to the cheek and forehead, but avoid putting pressure on the eyeball.
4. Go to the casualty department of the nearest hospital at once.

Retinal detachment

This condition is due to a number of causes, not necessarily injury, but I deal with it here as injury is one of the preventable ones. The light-sensitive retina lining the inside of the back of your eyes can become detached, rather like wallpaper peeling away from a wall. When this happens the detached part of the retina no longer functions. Retinal detachment occurs because a hole or tear develops in the retina. This allows fluid to pass behind the retina, separating it from the other coats of the eye (see Chapter 1).

Who gets retinal detachments?   Detachment of the retina is a rare condition, occurring in only one person in 10,000 each year.

- It happens mainly between the ages of twenty and sixty and is rare in children and the very elderly. Men are twice as often affected as women.
- Two-thirds of retinal detachments happen to people who are short-sighted – the greater the short sight the more common is retinal detachment. This is because the retina of a short-sighted person is weaker and more liable to tear.
- Severe injury to the eye is a direct cause. This can follow either a blunt injury or a penetrating wound (see pages 87, 89), and may be immediate or develop gradually as I describe in the symptoms (below). If your eyes are prominent there is a higher risk of retinal detachment as they are more susceptible to injury.
- Relatively minor trauma such as a light blow may also cause a detachment in those who are short-sighted and have a weak retina.
- After cataract surgery (see Chapter 9) two people in every hundred develop a retinal detachment.

The symptoms of retinal detachment

At least one-third of people get some advance warning of a retinal detachment. This is most commonly in the form of flashes of light which appear on the edge of the field of vision. These may be bright enough to be seen during daylight as well as at night. The description of the flashes varies from being 'like someone switching a light on and off' to sparks, arcs or flickers of light.

They may happen for short intervals or all the time, or you may notice them only as you move your eyes in one particular direction. We all tend to see spots before our eyes at some time, but the sudden appearance of a large number of small dots or a clouding of the sight may be a warning of a retinal detachment. Warning signs may occur for a month or longer before the symptoms of the retinal detachment appear.

There is no pain or discomfort when the detachment happens, the only symptom being a change in vision. A shadow or grey curtain appears on the edge of your field of vision and may spread rapidly to involve the central vision. When this occurs it is no longer possible to see to read. Occasionally there may be a shimmering appearance as if you are looking through water.

Treatment   A retinal detachment can be treated only by operation, which is usually performed under a general anaesthetic. The retina is repositioned by pieces of silicone rubber sponge being sewn to the outside of the back of the eye. Cryotherapy, which involves applying a freezing probe, then seals the retinal hole and sticks the retina to the other coats of the eye. This can be carried out under either general or local anaesthetic.

At least 80 per cent of retinal detachment operations are successful. However, if the detachment is particularly complicated it may be necessary to operate more than once.

After the operation   You will probably be able to sit out of bed on the day after the operation and will go home after about one week. You must move about cautiously to begin with, but you can return to sedentary work in six weeks. It will be four or five months before you can return to a properly active life.

Chemical injuries

These are not common but they require instant action. The speed that you start first aid treatment will determine the eventual effect on your sight.

Causes: in the home   You will almost certainly have weak chemical solutions as cleaners and disinfectants. Many of them are in pressurized containers that can easily be misdirected. In the garden chemical sprays are a source of damage to the eyes.

At work   The chemicals used in industry are often concentrated and the damage done by the eyes being splashed with them can be considerable. Lime used by builders in mortar or whitewash or cement is also very caustic to the eyes.

Treatment

The most important thing is speed. The aim is to dilute and wash out the chemical so that the time that it is in contact with the eye is kept to a minimum.

The best way to do this is with water, either under a running tap or by putting the person's head in a bucket or basin. If you don't have any water use the first available bland liquid such as milk, tea or water from a soda siphon. If there are any solid particles, especially lime, try to remove them.

After you have made every attempt to wash the eyes go to the nearest place that can give treatment. This is usually the casualty department of your local hospital.

Radiation injuries

Radiation is a very rare cause of injury. I see perhaps 10 cases each year. There are various possible sources, from exposure to X-rays or ultraviolet radiation to the visible radiation from the sun, or the invisible radiation following an atomic explosion. Of these, ultraviolet radiation burns are the most common.

Ultraviolet light radiation

The three common sources of ultraviolet radiation that can cause eye problems are:

1. Reflection of light from snow or water
2. Arc welding equipment
3. Sunray lamps.

The effects are the same, regardless of the source. Several hours after exposure your eyes feel extremely gritty and water profusely. It becomes increasingly difficult to open them due to spasm of the eyelid muscles, and any light causes marked discomfort.

The symptoms will settle without treatment within forty-eight hours as the damaged surface of the eyes heal. You should seek medical advice: you will need pain-killing tablets and should then go to bed with both eyes covered.

You may also ease the discomfort by applying cold compresses to your closed eyelids. Use a handkerchief soaked in cold water.

Eclipse burn

If you are foolish enough to look at the sun you may burn the back of your eye, in the same way that you can burn a leaf by concentrating the sun's rays with a magnifying glass: your eyes' lenses concentrate the rays inside your eyes. This injury has been given the name eclipse burn since so many people have damaged their eyes while gazing at an eclipse of the sun.

The results can be disastrous, with complete loss of your central vision, which is untreatable. Prevention is paramount. You should never look at the sun directly, even through smoked glass or over-exposed photographic film. If you must watch an eclipse of the sun, do so by making a pinhole in a piece of card and projecting the image of the sun on to black paper.

Never look directly at the sun when it is rising or setting, or even at its reflection in water or on glass.

Prevention of eye injuries

It is astonishing how many times I have heard the phrase, 'If only I had . . .' This is most often from the person who has suffered an accident, but occasionally it expresses a parent's regret at lack of supervision. To save you this anguish here are some of the 'if only' situations to avoid.

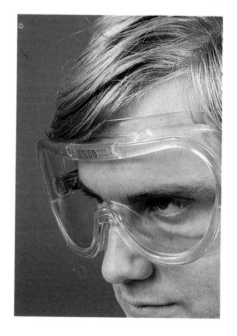

Always wear goggles to protect your eyes from possible injury in work or gardening.

Children

You can't watch them all the time but at least make sure that they don't have toys that are potentially dangerous. Bows with sharp arrows, and pistols that fire even plastic bullets, are fun but risky in the wrong hands.

Fireworks take an annual toll each year in the UK on 5th November and similar events in other countries. Fortunately their rising cost means they they are beyond the pockets of many children, and the trend towards well-organized parties supervised by adults has meant a marked drop in firework injuries. However, among those that are injured the eyes are most commonly involved.

Prevention at home

The best protection for your eyes is to wear protective glasses or goggles. This may not be possible for every dangerous activity but even when you don't use them, you should be particularly cautious with the following:

1. Household chemicals
2. Hammering – especially if you are using a cold chisel or old, worn tools
3. Electric power tools – especially when you are drilling, grinding, sawing or sanding.

Gardening

Wear protective goggles, even if they are uncomfortable in hot weather, for:

1. Rotary mowing
2. Hedge cutting with power-driven tools
3. Chopping wood
4. Power sawing
5. Creosote painting or spraying chemicals.

Driving

The following hints may save not only your eyesight but also your life:

1. Wear a properly adjusted seat belt.
2. Choose a laminated windscreen when buying a new car. Toughened safety glass tends to shatter into numerous small fragments that can injure your eyes.
3. Beware of elasticated luggage holders which hook on to a roof rack. Have someone else help hook the ends on.

Sports

There is fortunately an increasing tendency to wear eye protection for sports, but many people are still reluctant to use it as they find that it interferes with their vision. You should adjust to wearing protection if you play an active sport regularly.

1. Wear a protective visor for games such as cricket and squash.
2. If you wear glasses choose plastic lenses.
3. Consider wearing contact lenses instead of glasses.
4. Beware of fish hooks, especially when casting.

Work

If your job is at all dangerous and you are supplied with protective goggles, wear them. For welding you should wear tinted goggles, the density depending on the equipment you are using. If none are supplied insist that they are provided.

Do not remove protective guards from machinery just to make your work easier to see.

Although there are probably many other examples that you can think of or may have had the misfortune to experience, these are among the commonest dangers. If you follow the advice in the last part of this chapter, then I hope you will never need to say, 'If only I had . . .'

11 DISEASES THAT CAN AFFECT YOUR EYES

While most illnesses have little or no lasting effect on your eyesight, a few harm your vision and for these you will need specialist treatment for your eyes as well as the general condition.

Diabetes

Diabetes is a condition where your body is unable to produce enough insulin and so cannot break down your foods normally. As a result the amount of sugar in your blood increases. This in turn can damage your eyes, kidneys, nerves and blood vessels.

People who develop diabetes when young are usually insulin-dependent – needing injections of insulin to control their condition – while those who develop it in middle age can often be controlled with strict diet and may need pills. The longer you have had diabetes, the more likely you are to get the more serious eye problems, though specialists are now saying that even juvenile-onset diabetics may be able to avoid these if their diabetes is kept under strict control.

Testing
If you are found to have diabetes your doctor or specialist should see that your eyes are checked regularly for any changes. These can happen to the blood vessels inside your eyes, so besides the usual vision test you will have the inside of your eyes examined and possibly photographed for the doctor's records.

It is possible to see more detail of the blood vessels inside your eyes if they contain dye. To achieve this you will be given an injection of fluorescein dye into a vein in your arm. As the dye circulates in your bloodstream it passes to the eyes within seconds. Then a rapid series of photographs will be taken to show the dye filling the blood vessels.

The dye, which is yellow, tends to give the skin a yellowish or sunburnt appearance. This fades completely over several hours and the dye passes out of your body in the urine.

The main eye problems that you can get with diabetes are:

1. Blurred vision
2. Double vision

3. Cataracts
4. Sudden loss of sight.

Blurred vision

This affects most people with diabetes at some time and may remain just a minor problem. You notice it when diabetes develops, and it may in fact be the first sign that you have diabetes. The increase in your blood sugar makes you short-sighted by altering the power of the lens in your eye.

You should have your eyes tested. Your doctor will give you the normal vision test (see Chapter 3) and may find the changes of diabetes in the retina when examining the inside of your eye.

Blurring of vision that is caused by the onset of diabetes usually rights itself when the diabetes is controlled.

Blurring of the central area of your vision can also occur when you have had diabetes for some years. This is caused by changes in your light-sensitive retina that will be seen by your doctor when you are examined. You will need specialist treatment for this condition (see page 98).

Double vision

This is caused by weakness of one of the muscles that move your eyes so that one eye moves more than the other and you see double. For example, you may wake up and see two bedside lamps where there should be one. The double images may be side by side or one above the other, depending on which muscle is affected.

You should consult your doctor so that your eyes can be tested, but fortunately the weakness usually settles without treatment over a period of several weeks as the muscles and nerves in your eyes recover. During this time it will help if you wear a patch over one eye to prevent the double vision. You should not attempt to drive.

Cataracts

Cataracts develop in diabetics in the same way as in non-diabetics and are about as common. Your specialist will be keeping a check on your eyes and will know when a cataract starts to develop. (For treatment see Chapter 9.)

Sudden loss of sight

The most troublesome of all the diabetic eye changes affect the light-sensitive retina and it is mainly to check for these that your specialist will give you regular eye tests. Two-thirds of all those who have had diabetes for twenty years or more have some retinal changes, but the majority have no problems with seeing. Only one in ten suffers from serious complications that require treatment. This may not restore perfect sight but it will prevent further deterioration.

You may notice the sudden appearance of dark spots or streaks that are caused by bleeding inside your eye. If this is severe your vision may be completely obscured. It is due to a weakening of the blood vessels which leak blood into the retina or into the vitreous fluid that fills the space between the retina and your lens.

Treatment   Small amounts of blood can be absorbed without treatment, but if you have more extensive bleeding you may need to be admitted to hospital for complete rest. If the rest does not clear the blood, you can have surgery to remove it.

Changes in the retina that are found in time can be treated very successfully with photocoagulation by laser beam. This involves using a very bright light to burn a small area of retina and shut off the leaking blood vessels.

You need only attend hospital as an outpatient for this procedure, which can be carried out using a local anaesthetic given as eyedrops. The sensation is similar to looking at repeated photographic flashes. As many as 2000 flashes of light may be given at a single session. Although this sounds extreme it is not, in fact. You will be very dazzled afterwards though and should have someone to accompany you home. Any discomfort that you may notice after the treatment usually wears off within several hours.

The results of this type of treatment are very dramatic, and the retinal changes may even completely disappear. Although this may not produce any improvement in your vision it will remove the cause of the bleeding which threatens your sight. It may be necessary to have several sessions of treatment to produce a satisfactory result. Afterwards you will need to attend for regular check-ups. Occasionally further treatment will be given if new changes are found in your eyes.

How can you as a diabetic avoid eye troubles?
The most important way that you can help yourself is by making sure that your diabetes is well controlled, for if the sugar levels in your blood fluctuate from day to day your sight will vary as well.

There is a tendency for the new diabetic to be meticulous with the control of the disease. As the years pass this careful approach is replaced by an easygoing attitude that may become indifference. Don't let this happen to you. With good control of the disease not only will you reduce the risk of eye problems, but you will also diminish the changes of diabetes affecting the rest of your body.

High blood pressure

High blood pressure is most commonly discovered when your doctor tests your blood pressure in the course of a general examination. However, it may also be found during a routine test for glasses when the specialist will see changes in the size and shape of the blood vessels at the back of your eyes.

The great majority of people who have high blood pressure do not notice any problems with their eyes. For a few, one of the following symptoms may be the first sign that the blood pressure is too high:

1. Double vision
2. Spots in your vision
3. Blurring of vision.

Double vision

Double vision can occur with raised blood pressure in the same way as it does in diabetes (see page 97).

There is no special treatment and usually your vision becomes normal again within six weeks. A patch worn over one eye overcomes the double vision. You should not attempt to drive, even when wearing a patch, as your assessment of distance and speed are severely affected.

Spots in your vision

Bleeding in the eyes tends to occur in people with high blood pressure over sixty. In this case the sudden appearance of spots or streaks in your vision is caused by blood leaking from the retinal vessels at the back of your eye – again, as in diabetes. If the bleeding is severe your sight will first become hazy all over and then be completely obscured.

You should see your family doctor who will test your eyes to ensure you do not have any other similar eye problems. Otherwise no special treatment is necessary, but you must rest as much as possible. Avoid any strenuous activities that may cause further bleeding.

Very rarely, if there has been no improvement in the sight after six months, an operation to remove the blood may be necessary.

Blurring of vision

Blurring of the top or bottom of your vision is caused by a blockage in either an artery or a vein in your retina. This is different from the blurred vision you get with other conditions such as cataract when the sight fails gradually. There are also different effects depending on whether an artery or a vein is blocked:

- With a vein you will just notice a vague blurring of the upper or lower part of your vision.
- If an artery is blocked, it will seem as if a shutter or curtain has suddenly been drawn across your vision either from above or below.
- The loss of vision may be complete if either the main or central retinal artery or vein becomes blocked.

It is important to seek medical attention as soon as possible. When an artery is involved every minute matters, and the earlier that treatment can be started the greater the chance of recovering your sight. Unfortunately it is often hours or even days before advice is sought, by which time it is too late.

When the main artery is affected there is less than a fifty-fifty chance of recovering any sight. When the blockage is in a vein the long-term effects are not so serious. After several weeks the vision gradually returns and there can be a full recovery after three months.

In those with the central vein blocked about one-third improve, one-third remain unchanged and one-third gradually lose vision.

Treatment   For a blockage in the main artery you will be admitted to hospital. Massage may be given to your eye and possibly pressure-reducing drugs (see page 66). When the vein is affected you may be given pills to help the flow of blood, but time and patience are usually all that are needed.

Once your vision is restored or the deterioration has been halted, there need be no restrictions on your normal activities.

A complication: thrombotic glaucoma

Approximately 10 per cent of people with obstruction of the main retinal vein also develop a type of glaucoma called thrombotic glaucoma. This will be discovered during the first three months following treatment and can be treated with the laser beam (see page 98) or by pressure-reducing drugs. The results are not always good, though, and your vision never returns to normal.

Headaches

One less common effect of having high blood pressure is recurring head-aches. These tend to be bad in the morning, gradually improving during the day. The condition known as migraine can be far more severe and if you are a sufferer you will know how your vision is dramatically affected and how bad the headaches that you may get in an attack can be. Because your sight is involved, I shall deal briefly with the condition here, although migraine is really a general health problem rather than an eye ailment. For more detailed advice on coping with migraine you can read *Migraine and Headaches* by Marcia Wilkinson, also in this series.

Migraine

Migraine affects as many as one in ten of the population, from small children to the elderly. It most commonly occurs from the teens to about

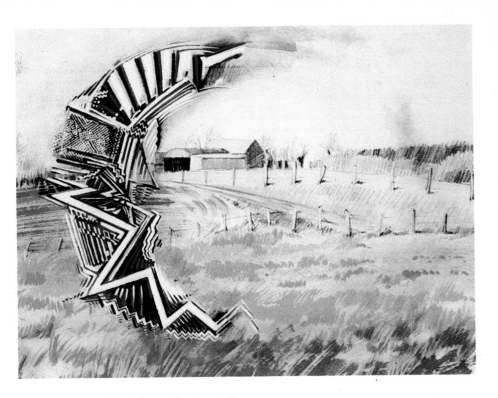

Visual effects, painted by a migraine sufferer.

the age of fifty. Women are three times more likely to be affected than men. Migraine may take one of three forms:

1. Classical migraine
2. Common or simple migraine
3. Migrainous neuralgia.

The same person may suffer one, two or even all three types at different times in their life. It is quite common for a teenager who suffers from classical migraine to change later to the common variety.

A classical migraine attack begins with a disturbance of the senses, called the aura. Your vision is most often affected, but the sense of feeling in an arm or leg and occasionally hearing and balance may also be upset.

Your first attack of migraine can be quite frightening because of the sudden upset in your vision, so that you may find difficulty in describing exactly what did happen. Flashing lights appear in the side vision of one or both eyes. These appear like rainbow-coloured sparks or flashes of lightning. Within a few minutes the area of the lights gradually expands and may fill all but the central part of your vision. Sometimes the reverse happens, with a central bright or blank spot becoming larger. The spot is

101

edged by a zigzag pattern of coloured lights which by expanding eventually reach the extreme edges of your vision and disappear.

The flashing lights usually last up to half an hour, but the central patch of blank vision may last longer and take several hours to recover.

Common migraine is a typical headache on one side without the flashing lights but with nausea and vomiting. Occasionally you may get the visual changes of classical migraine without the headache.

Migrainous neuralgia is a very unusual form of migraine that affects four times as many men as women. You get bouts of headache over several weeks which may wake you at night. The headache tends to be centred around one eye, and this may water and become red. The pain may spread down the side of your nose and the nostril on that side may become blocked.

Treatment of migraine

1. While the attack is on, lie down in a darkened room.
2. You should see your doctor if you have any of these types of migraine. A drug treatment will probably be prescribed, or tablets that can be bought over the counter recommended.
3. Try and ward off further attacks by avoiding the foods and situations that seem to start the migraine.
4. Learning methods of relaxation can help you deal with the attacks.

Why it is important to recognize migraine

Migraine can cause changes in your sight that may be similar to the ones that several eye troubles produce, such as floaters or the more serious problem of the light-sensitive retina (see Chapter 10). After you have recovered from a migraine attack your eyes return to normal so that your doctor will find nothing to help in making a diagnosis. It is therefore important to try to notice exactly what happens to your vision and for how long. Imagine that you will have to write down the changes and you will then be able to describe them more accurately and so help your doctor separate migraine from other diseases.

Floaters

It is very common for people of any age to see small spots or floaters. They are caused by a change in the consistency of the vitreous fluid between your lens and retina (see Chapter 1). Floaters take on many forms from small dots or threads to the very life-like appearance of spiders, flies or even tadpoles. They may appear so clear that you can draw their shape exactly. They move with your eye movements and tend to swing back and forth across your vision.

There is no treatment for them and other than their nuisance value you needn't worry about them as they do not usually signify eye disease.

If, however, they appear at the same time as you see flashes of light you should consult your doctor, since you may have some weakness of your retina (see page 90) which needs treatment, or a haemorrhage due to high blood pressure or diabetes (see pages 97, 99).

Strokes

A stroke is a disturbance of the function of the brain caused either by blockage in a blood vessel or bleeding from a weakened blood vessel. There is a sudden partial or complete loss of consciousness together with weakness of the muscles of one side of the body so that movements of the arm and leg are affected. Only about one in ten who have had a stroke are severely disabled.

Sight may be affected after a stroke either due to damage to the nerves passing from the eyes so that the brain can't see, or to the brain not recognizing what it can see. If the speech is affected too the person is unable to explain what he or she can or can't see.

How strokes affect vision

Four out of five strokes occur because of interruption of the blood supply to the brain due to thrombosis – blood clot formation.

The brain is divided into two halves or hemispheres, each with its own blood supply. Each hemisphere is responsible for the sensation and movement of the opposite half of the body. It also serves the vision for the opposite side. Therefore, the left hemisphere not only moves the right side of the body but also sees everything on the right side of the vision in each eye, while the right hemisphere moves the left side of the body and sees everything on the left of the vision in each eye (see page 104).

So if there is loss of vision from a stroke it always affects both eyes. A variable amount of the left or right side of the field of vision in either eye is lost. When the loss is over a large part of the field of vision people and objects are missed, making day-to-day chores difficult.

Strokes affecting vision also make reading a problem. If the loss is on the right side it is impossible to read across a line of print. When the left side is affected people often complain that they lose their place when reading because they cannot find the beginning of the next line of print. You can't do anything about the right-sided loss, but when the left side is affected you can use your finger as a marker. If your left hand is also weak you have to use your right hand.

Treatment

There is no medical treatment for strokes. Recovery depends on the severity of the stroke, the concentration of the patient and

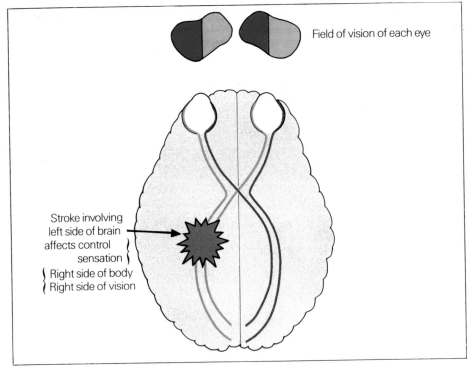

Field of vision of each eye

Stroke involving
left side of brain
affects control
sensation
Right side of body
Right side of vision

The effects on vision of a stroke (eyes and brain seen from above).

determination to improve. These are often missing in the elderly and so the recognition of visual problems by relatives and medical staff are important for successful rehabilitation.

TIAs

Some strokes are preceded by short episodes of weakness or loss of sensation in an arm or leg, difficulty with speech and impaired vision, lasting from a few minutes to several hours. These are caused by a temporary loss of blood supply to the brain or eyes and are called transient ischaemic attacks (TIAs).

The effect on the sight is to produce a sudden painless loss of vision in one eye like a curtain coming down. It lasts for only two to three minutes, after which there is a gradual recovery to normal. Because the effects on the rest of the body are equally short-lived they are sometimes only noticed by other people.

Treatment   It is extremely important to have treatment for TIAs as without it there is a strong likelihood of you suffering a major stroke within five years – in fact a 30 to 50 per cent chance.

Treatment is with anticoagulant drugs to help reduce the clotting of the blood. Occasionally it is possible to operate on narrowed arteries in the neck which are sites of clot formation.

Other troubles: thyroid disorders

The thyroid gland that lies in the neck in front of the windpipe or trachea helps maintain the normal metabolism of the body.

The commonest upset is over-activity of the gland causing the condition called thyrotoxicosis or hyperthyroidism. The most noticeable feature of this is the alteration in the appearance of the eyes, which appear more prominent than normal, with more of the white of the eye showing. There is often some redness and the eyes feel gritty. The tissues behind the eyes swell and cause the enlarged look, as well as weakening the eye muscles. This may result in a squint and double vision, as the eyes do not move together. In very severe cases pressure on the optic nerve may damage the sight.

Treatment for the eyes is as follows:

With hyperthyroidism, the eyes become prominent, with more of the white of the eye showing.

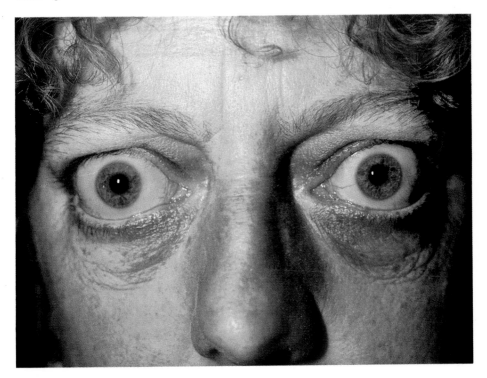

1. Eyedrops will be prescribed to help lubricate the exposed front of the eyes, with ointment to be used at night.
2. If you have double vision you will need to wear an eye patch.
3. An operation to correct a squint may be necessary if double vision persists for longer than six to nine months (see Chapter 7).
4. The widening of the eyelids can be overcome in some people by using eyedrops or by an operation to join the outer thirds of the upper and lower lids.
5. If your sight is threatened due to pressure on the optic nerve, corticosteroid pills and possibly surgery will be needed.

Retinitis pigmentosa

Retinitis pigmentosa is the name given to a rare group of hereditary eye diseases that affect the retina. These are sometimes part of a condition involving other areas of the body too. Retinitis pigmentosa results in a progressive loss of vision. Reports in the popular press have brought publicity with extravagant claims of cures ranging from bee stings to acupuncture and from placental implants to hormone injections. There is unfortunately no real evidence that any of these methods is effective.

The symptoms, which affect both eyes, are night blindness or difficulty in seeing in dim light, and loss of the side vision. The loss of side vision may progress until only a small central area of sight remains (tunnel vision). This central island of vision may last until the age of sixty or seventy, but occasionally it may be lost with the development of a cataract. The effect of tunnel vision is to make the person appear clumsy as he or she bumps into unseen furniture or trips on steps.

How does it develop?

Symptoms usually begin around the age of ten and can be quite marked by the age of twenty. The course of the loss of vision is slow and varies between individuals and the different types of the disease. There may be long periods with no deterioration and occasions when the sight may even improve. It is probably these periods of remission that explain the apparent success of the miracle cures that falsely raise people's hopes.

Treatment

1. Anyone with retinitis pigmentosa should see a genetic specialist. You should supply a detailed history of other affected members of your family to help decide which type of the disease you have and what is likely to happen to your vision. You will also be given advice about the chances of your children being affected.
2. Although there is no known cure to restore or even preserve sight, it is possible with low vision aids (see Chapter 9) and correct lighting for you to use your remaining vision.

3. You may need cataract surgery (see above and Chapter 9). This can produce dramatic improvement in vision for some people.
4. In the United Kingdom there is an active society of people with retinitis pigmentosa whose aims are to help overcome the visual handicap and to raise funds for research. Similar societies exist in Europe, North America and Australia (see the Useful Addresses section at the end of this book).

Multiple sclerosis

This is an uncommon condition. It affects the normal working of the nerves and some parts of the brain. It develops between the ages of twenty and forty and is slightly more common in women than men. The cause is unknown, but while it occurs in Europe and Britain it is less common in North America and rare in the Middle East, Africa, India and Japan. It is a peculiar condition as episodes of trouble are often followed by long periods when the person has no problems.

One-third of all sufferers notice difficulties with vision as the first sign of the disease. Other general problems are difficulty with moving the legs, disturbances of the sense of touch and slurring of the speech.

The eye problems

1. Blurring of the vision in one eye happens to over 50 per cent of people with MS at some time. As one optic nerve becomes affected there is a period of three or four days when the eyeball is tender and it hurts to look upwards. This is followed by the blurring of vision. Fortunately your eyesight recovers completely over several weeks without treatment.

   Brief blurring of vision is sometimes noticed with physical exertion or if you take a very hot bath.
2. You may notice double vision for periods of up to a few days to several weeks, but this usually disappears without treatment.
3. In over 60 per cent of people with multiple sclerosis there is a jerky movement of the eyes from side to side. It does not affect the sight.

The prospects for the multiple sclerosis patient

There is a great tendency for anyone who is diagnosed as suffering from multiple sclerosis to assume that it is only a matter of time before he or she is confined to a wheelchair and unable to move. Although there are inevitably a few severely disabled sufferers the majority are able to live normal lives.

The first attack of eye trouble may be your only attack, while for others there may be no further problems for at least twenty years. The popular belief that the diagnosis of multiple sclerosis is a sentence for you to be treated as an invalid is quite wrong.

12 LIVING WITH YOUR FAILING SIGHT

The shock of being told that there is no cure may, at first, make battling against the daily problems in a world dependent on normal sight seem pointless. You tend to think that poor vision like other ailments only happens to other people. This is a natural reaction, for while we accept the changes of growing old, we may also secretly feel that we enjoy a certain immunity to protect us from everybody else's ills.

Coming to terms with failing sight is difficult at any age although some people adapt more easily than others. In this chapter I want to show how best you can manage, either for yourself or a member of your family. There is plenty of help available from organizations and groups both for partially sighted and blind people (see the Useful Addresses section) and you should not hesitate to contact these. Being in touch with people in the same position as yourself can be a great encouragement.

How to cope with partial sight
It is important to make the most of whatever sight you may have. In this chapter I intend to give as much positive help on these lines as limited space allows. Some of the advice appears in other chapters and for this I make no apology as it cannot be over-emphasized.

Lighting   Your vision in daylight will be better than under artificial light. Colours are easier to distinguish, and so you should try to do your sewing, embroidery or painting during the day. If you are using artificial lighting make sure it is bright enough and that it is in the correct position, that is, shining directly over your shoulder from just behind your head.

Light shining directly on your eyes causes dazzle, so out of doors wear a hat with a brim or an eye-shield, and in general keep your eyes protected from direct lighting.

Make sure that the lighting all around your house is good, not just in the main living areas. Hallways and stairs are often dimly lit and are potential hazards for those with a visual handicap.

If you are in strange surroundings and you think your vision has suddenly got worse stop and decide if it is the lighting that is at fault.

Contrast
• Telephone numbers are often difficult to read, especially the figures 3, 5 and 8 that all appear similar. It will help if you get someone to make

a list of the numbers that you often use with a black felt-tipped pen.
- Large print telephone numbers printed on a label to fit over the telephone dial will help.
- Ask friends and relatives writing to you to use a felt-tipped pen.
- If you have difficulty seeing food on a dark plate, use a plain but lighter coloured plate.
- If there are steps around your home, have a white line painted along the front edge of the tread of each step.

Glasses
- Make sure that you are wearing the right glasses for the distance you are trying to view. Elderly people often get confused and may try to look at the television set with their reading glasses.
- Tinted lenses may help in some conditions, for example, if you have cataracts or retinitis pigmentosa.

Low vision aids There are various LVAs that will be recommended by your specialist if they will help you. These I describe on page 83.

Large print books As a result of the success of the Ulverscroft series there are now several British and American publishers producing large print books. These are usually only available through public libraries although some of the reference books like dictionaries can also be bought. Although the choice of large print books is limited these books have enabled many people to continue the pleasure of reading despite their failing sight.

Living with a visual handicap
There is an ever-increasing number of clubs, societies and groups to help the visually handicapped, so there should be no shortage of people who are able and very willing to give time and advice. In the UK the main body is the Royal National Institute for the Blind (RNIB) and around the world there are similar organizations such as the American Foundation for the Blind, the Canadian National Institute for the Blind, the Royal New Zealand Foundation for the Blind and several state institutes in Australia.

In the United Kingdom there is a weekly BBC Radio broadcast called 'In Touch' made and presented by blind broadcasters and journalists. There is also a BBC publication called *In Touch* which contains a wealth of advice to visually handicapped people and their relatives. This book can be bought from BBC Publications and is a must for the relatives of any visually handicapped person. A braille edition is also available.

In North America and Australia special radio programmes are broadcast for blind listeners by many radio stations.

Registration
When your vision has reached a certain level your specialist will suggest you register so that you can benefit from a variety of services provided free or at a low cost.

If you are not already being seen by an eye specialist but are having trouble with your sight you can apply to be registered. You should consult your family doctor, who will send you to a specialist for a test to decide whether you should be registered.

In either case, you will be tested to determine whether you should be registered as partially sighted or blind.

The partially sighted person can usually only read the top half of the distance vision chart; but even if the central vision is better than this, he or she may still be registered if the side vision is restricted.

Registration as blind does not imply that you have no sight. The definition in the UK is 'that a person should be so blind as to be unable to perform any work for which eyesight is essential'.

Why register?
You may feel there is a stigma attached to being registered, but I hope you will realize as you read this chapter that the advantages far outweigh your early doubts.

Registration alerts the local social services to the problems of the visually handicapped person: for a child steps will be taken to ensure that proper schooling is continued; for those who are below retirement age, a course of retraining for a different job can be recommended so that they may return to some form of employment. The majority of people registered are retired, and they often suffer other handicaps as well as loss of sight. As the social services learn about this, aid can be given for these other problems too.

All the support for the visually handicapped that I describe below will be available once you have registered. As your sight gets worse, you will experience more difficulty in daily routines that used to be automatic. The assistance of the social services in learning new techniques will be invaluable.

Getting about
Learning to get around not only in your own home, but also in the outside world is a major hurdle for the newly visually handicapped. In the United Kingdom after you have been registered blind the local social service department arranges a visit from a mobility officer to teach you how to manage.

White cane   You will be shown how to use a white cane as a guide. This

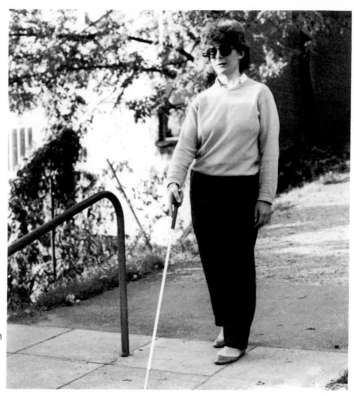

A white cane is both a guide for a blind person and a sign to others.

does not provide the support of a normal walking stick but acts as a guide for yourself and a sign to other people.

The most useful way of getting around is by the long cane method. You swing the cane from side to side as you take each step forward. The sensitive, light cane will touch any obstruction and give you an idea of changes in levels. It may take several months to master this technique, but with it you will be able to get around quickly and with confidence.

Rather than using the long cane some people keep a guide cane or symbol stick to use in a crowded place.

Guide dogs   A guide dog is only suitable for a small percentage of blind people since the owner has to be physically fit to ensure that the dog is exercised regularly.

In the UK those people who feel that they would like a guide dog are interviewed by representatives of the Guide Dog Association. If they are accepted a four week residential course is arranged at one of the five special training centres.

Electronic aids   There are various aids that use inaudible ultrasound beams

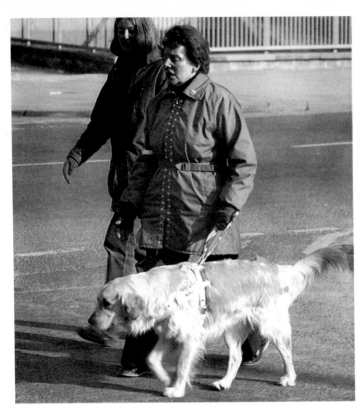

For the physically fit blind person, a guide dog is a great help and companion.

to identify obstacles. The ultrasound waves are converted into audible sounds in headphones or into vibrations in hand-held instruments. These aids are expensive and rather difficult to use. I would only recommend one as an extra to the white cane or guide dog.

Communication

The problems for a blind person of keeping in touch can be considerable. The loss of independence that blindness brings can never be fully overcome. You will always have to rely on someone else to read a letter or fill in a form. But by learning new skills you will be able to read and write. Many visually handicapped people have useful and satisfying jobs and enjoy plenty of hobbies and pastimes once they have mastered the new techniques.

Reading

Braille is the best known method. The originator, Louis Braille, devised a code of raised dots to represent the letters of the alphabet and punctuation signs (see opposite) which can be read by touch. The method is very adaptable and can also be used for mathematics, scientific purposes and music.

To learn to read braille requires determination and perseverance, but once you acquire the skill you have considerable self-sufficiency.

Moon type is an embossed alphabet and is useful if you find braille too difficult to master. The symbols are large, simplified versions of ordinary print (see below). The choice of books available in Moon print is smaller than for braille, but the method is particularly suitable for the elderly who find braille difficult to learn.

Optacon is a reading machine (*Optical Tactile Converter*). The print is 'read' by a small camera and is converted into a pattern that can be felt by one finger. The method allows you to read ordinary print at the rate of about thirty to forty words a minute.

Writing

If you want to continue writing in longhand you can use a writing frame to help keep you on a straight line, and a similar device can be used to sign

Examples of braille and Moon type alphabets.

BRAILLE ALPHABET

A	B	C	D	E	F	G	H	I	J

K	L	M	N	O	P	Q	R	S	T

GRADE 1 MOON

B	C	D	E	F	G	H	I	J
2	3	4	5	6	7	8	9	0

L	M	N	O	P	Q	R	S

U	V	W	X	Y	Z	AND	TH THE

113

cheques. Alternatively you can use a typewriter and this certainly repays the effort of learning.

While the writing produced by these methods can be read by sighted people it is very helpful for you to be able to write Braille as well. In this way you can make a note of an address or telephone number so that you will be able to find it again.

You imprint the dots on paper using either a hand frame that is small enough to carry in your pocket or a machine the size of a typewriter.

The main disadvantage of writing in Braille is that it takes up a large amount of paper. Instead you can use a small cassette recorder to store useful items.

Listening

Listening to the radio, television or recorded tapes is probably the most important way for visually handicapped people to keep in touch.

Radio and television   In the United Kingdom all registered blind people are entitled to a radio which is on free permanent loan. Blind people may also get a reduction on the licence for a television.

Talking Book Service   Tape recordings of a wide selection of books are available from the British Talking Book Service. The annual subscription, usually paid by your local authority, gives you access to nearly 4000 books with the sort of titles you will find in a public library ranging from the classics to the latest best-sellers.

The special large-sized cassettes have twelve hours of listening, but these can only be played on a machine loaned by the Talking Book Service. The cassettes are exchanged free by post.

In the United States the Library for the Blind and Physically Handicapped has an even larger selection of books; and both London and New York have Student Tape Libraries with cassette recordings of educational books.

Talking newspaper   In the United Kingdom the Talking Newspaper Association provides taped versions of many local newspapers. The cassettes can be played back on an ordinary cassette recorder. The tapes are exchanged by post each week or fortnight. In other countries there are similar agencies (see page 117).

Tape recording services   There are several services that will record material if requested. The charge is the price of a cassette. But if you send a blank tape the recording is usually free. There are also services for religious material and tape correspondence clubs. (For addresses of these services see pages 117–19.)

How to guide a blind person

While blindness produces sympathy from normally sighted people there is often a tendency to oversimplify conversation as if the person were a child, or to raise your voice rather like the caricatured Englishman abroad. Apart from a few elderly blind people who may have also become deaf and mentally inactive, the vast majority of visually handicapped people differ only in their loss of vision. Indeed some may have a greater awareness of their surroundings with sharper hearing and keener sense of touch than most of us. If you bear these points in mind you will be able to help and communicate with blind people in a way they appreciate most.

When meeting a blind person announce your presence, saying who you are.

During a group conversation always address a blind person by name. Otherwise he or she will not know when to join in. At the end, say if you are leaving to save the person the embarrassment of talking to thin air.

The correct way to guide a blind person.

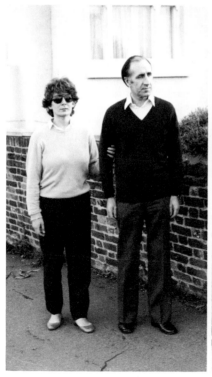
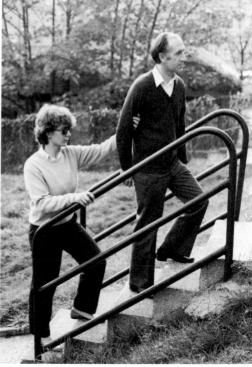

Guiding a blind person is simple when you know how, but is a skill that must be learned.

Walking   Don't take hold of the blind person's arm, but offer yours. He or she should hold it just above the elbow. In this way you lead the way with the blind person half a pace behind you. If you have to walk in single file, keep your arm straight at the middle of your back.

Doorways   Always approach a door with the blind person on the same side of you as the hinges. As you turn the handle using the arm that is being held the blind person will know if the door is opening inwards or outwards. When you have walked through the door the blind person can shut the door with his or her free hand.

Stairs   Use the same arm grip as for walking on the level (see above). Start by saying 'stairs up' or 'stairs down', then step on to the first step. The blind person will feel the upward or downward movement of your arm. He or she can then follow, moving in rhythm with you and one step behind you. When you reach the top or the bottom the change in position of your arm will be felt, so that the blind person knows there are no more steps.

Chairs   Use a similar technique to get a blind person into a chair: approach the chair centrally from the front, back or side and place your guiding hand on the back of the chair. Let your partner slide his or her hand down your arm to the chair and feel for the seat.

There is an enormous amount of help to be had from the special organizations that deal with your particular problem in your locality. If you do not have the address of the nearest branch, apply to the appropriate head office. I give the address of these on the next few pages.

USEFUL ADDRESSES

Note: For addresses of local independent organizations, ask your nearest national agency.

UNITED KINGDOM

Association for the Education and Welfare of the Visually Handicapped
East Anglian School
Church Road
Gorleston-on-Sea
Great Yarmouth
Norfolk
NR31 6LP

British National Committee for the Prevention of Blindness
191 Old Marylebone Road
London NW1 5QN

British Retinitis Pigmentosa Society
Hon Sec: Mrs L. M. Drummond-Walker
24 Palmer Close
Redhill
Surrey RH1 4BX

British Talking Service for the Blind
Mount Pleasant
Alperton
Wembley
Middlesex HA0 1RR

Electronic Aids for the Blind
28 Crofton Avenue
Orpington
Kent BR6 8DU

General Optical Council
41 Harley Street
London W1N 2DJ

Guide Dogs for the Blind Association
Alexandra House
9–11 Park Street
Windsor
Berkshire SL4 1JR

Institute of Ophthalmology
41 Judd Street
London WC1 9QS

National Federation of the Blind
45 South Street
Normanton
West Yorkshire
WF6 1EE

National Library for the Blind
Cromwell Road
Bredbury
Stockport
SK6 2SG

Optical Information Council
Walter House
418–22 The Strand
London WC2R 2PB

Partially Sighted Society
40 Wordsworth Street
Hove
East Sussex
BN3 5BH

Royal National Institute for the Blind
224 Great Portland Street
London W1N 6AA

Braille and Tape Libraries
Braille House
338 Goswell Road
London EC1

Scottish Braille Press
Craigmillar Park
Edinburgh
Lothian EH16 5NB

Talking Newspaper Association for the United Kingdom
c/o Mrs J. Deaper
4 Southgate Street
Winchester
Hants SO23 9EF

Tape Recording Service for the Blind
48 Fairfax Road
Farnborough
Hants GU14 8JF

Ulverscroft Large-Print Books
The Green
Bradgate Road
Anstey
Leicester LE7 7FU

UNITED STATES

American Foundation for the Blind
15 West 16th Street
New York, NY 10011

American Printing House for the Blind
1839 Frankfort Avenue
Louisville, KY 40206

Association for Macular Diseases
PO Box 469
Merrick, NY 11566

Better Vision Institute
230 Park Avenue
New York, NY 10017

Carroll Center for the Blind
770 Centre Street
Newton, MA 02158
(rehabilitation)

Library of Congress
National Library Service for the Blind
   and Physically Handicapped
1291 Taylor Street, NW
Washington, DC 20542

Myopia International Research
   Foundation
415 Lexington Avenue, Rm 705
New York, NY 10017

National Association of Optometrists
   and Opticians
18903 S Miles Road
Cleveland, OH 44128

National Association for the Visually
   Handicapped
305 East 24th Street, 17–C
New York, NY 10010

National Braille Association
422 Clinton Avenue South
Rochester, NY 14620

National Children's Eye Care
   Foundation
1101 Connecticut Avenue, NW,
   Suite 700
Washington, DC 20036

National Eye Institute
Information Office
National Institute of Health
Bldg 31, Rm 6A32
Bethesda, MD 20205

National Eye Research Foundation
18 S Michigan Avenue
Chicago, IL 60603

National Retinitis Pigmentosa
   Foundation
Rolling Park Bldg
8331 Mindale Circle
Baltimore, MD 21207

National Society for the Prevention of
   Blindness
79 Madison Avenue
New York, NY 10016

Public and Professional Education
   Committee
American Academy of Ophthalmology
PO Box 7424
San Francisco, CA 94120

Recording for the Blind
215 East 58th Street
New York, NY 10022

Volunteers for Vision
PO Box 2211
Austin, TX 78768
(children)

Low-cost eye examinations and
   eyeglasses are available at
New York University School of
   Optometry
100 East 24th Street
New York, NY 10010

and at most other optometry schools
   throughout the country

CANADA

Association of Canadian Optometrists
77 Metcalfe Street
Suite 207
Ottawa, ON
KIP 5L6

Association of Ontario Optometrists
40 St Clair Avenue West
Toronto, ON
M4V 1M2

Canadian Foundation for Disabled and Handicapped Persons
2057 Danforth Avenue
Toronto, ON
M4C 1J8

Canadian National Institute for the Blind
320 Mcleod Street
Ottawa, ON
K2P 1AE

Low Vision Association of Ontario
1 Dundas Street West
PO Box 10
Toronto, ON
M5G 1Z3

National Retina Pigmentosa Foundation of Canada
1 Spadina Crescent
Toronto, ON
M5S 2J5

Optometric Institute of Toronto
815 Danford Avenue
Suite 301
Toronto, ON
M4J 1L2

AUSTRALIA

Australian Federation of Blind Citizens
18 Albert Avenue
Tranmere
SA 5073

Australian National Council for the Blind
7 Mair Street
Brighton Beach
Victoria 3188

119

ACKNOWLEDGEMENTS

I would like to thank my secretaries Jennie Harvey and Lynne Smith for typing the manuscripts, Kay Deakin for her many helpful suggestions and Mary Banks for patiently guiding the editing.

1984   MICHAEL GLASSPOOL

The publishers are grateful to the following for their help in the preparation of this book:
For reading and commenting on the manuscript: David Harrisberg, Dip Optom (SA).
For permission to reproduce photographs: the ARCO Group, Hull (page 93); Pictor International, London (page 69); RNIB, London (page 112); and WB Pharmaceuticals, Bracknell (page 101).
The cover and photographs on pages 28, 32, 53, 76, 77 and 88 were modelled by Gillian Walker and taken by Roland Kemp. The white cane was kindly lent by the RNIB and the furniture and other props by the Reject Shop, London.
The diagrams were drawn by David Gifford.

INTERNATIONAL DRUG NAME EQUIVALENTS

Generic name	Great Britain Trade name	Australia Trade name
atropine	Isopto Atropine	Atropt
neomycin	Myciguent (ointment) (drops available only in combination with other ingredients)	Neopt
sodium cromoglycate	Opticrom	Opticrom
adrenaline	Eppy; Epifrin; Isopto Epinal	Epinal; Epifrin; Eppy/N; Glaucon
pilocarpine	Isopto Carpine; Sno-Pilo	Isopto Carpine; Neutracarpine; Pilopt
guanethidine	Ismelin; Ganda	not available as eye preparations
acetazolamide	Diamox	Glaucomide; Diamox
timolol	Timoptol	Timoptol
dichlorphenamide	Daranide; Oratrol	Daranide

Generic name	United States Trade name	Canada Trade name
atropine	Isopto Atropine; Atropisol	Isopto Atropine
neomycin	Myciguent (ointment) (drops available only in combination with other ingredients)	not available as eye preparations
cromolyn sodium (sodium cromoglycate)	not available as eye preparations	Opticrom
epinephrine	Epifrin; Glaucon; Epitrate	Epinal; Glaucon; Epifrin
pilocarpine	Isopto Carpine; Almocarpine; Pilomiotin	Isopto Carpine; P.V. Carpine
guanethidine	not available as eye preparations	not available as eye preparations
acetazolamide	Diamox	Acetazolam; Diamox
timolol	Timoptic	Timoptic
dichlorphenamide	Daranide; Oratrol	not available

INDEX

Page numbers in *italic* refer to the illustrations.

glasses, 33–41; *40*; after cataract
surgery, 79–80; failing sight, 109;
frames, 37–8; lenses, 38–40; low
vision aids, 83–4; *83*; myths, 28; for
squints, 61; tests, 36–7; tinted lenses,
40–1
glaucoma, 50, 54, 63–72; *64*; acute,
70–1; children, 56, 72; chronic,
63–70; diagnosis, 19, 65; secondary,
71–2; symptoms, 14, 16, 21, 64–5;
thrombotic, 100
guanethidine, 66, 67, 68
guide dogs, 111; *112*
guiding the blind, 115–16; *115*

half vision, 13, 15
hay fever, 16, 42, 46–7
headaches, 15, 16, 100
herpes simplex, 48, 49, 50
high blood pressure, 15, 24, 98–100,
103
hyperthyroidism, 105; *105*

injuries, 85–95
iris, 9, 10, 70, 87
iritis, 14, 16, 48, 50–1, 72

jaundice, 17

keratoconus, 49

lazy eyes, 60–1
lenses (eye), 9, 10; cataract, 73–4,
77–8; lens implants, 81–2
lenses: contact lenses, 41–3; glasses,
38–41; *40*; low vision aids, 83–4; *83*
lighting, for reading, 75–6, 108; *76, 77*
long sight, 33–4, 41, 55, 59; *34*
loss of vision, 13–15; diabetes, 97;
glaucoma, 65; retinitis pigmentosa,
106; strokes, 103; *104*; TIAs, 104
low vision aids (LVAs), 83–4, 109; *83*

macula, 10; degeneration of, 82–4
migraine, 15, 100–2; *101*
Moon type, 113; *113*
multifocal lenses, 39; *40*
multiple sclerosis, 15, 107
muscles, of the eye, 23, 29, 59–60, 86,
97, 105; *see also* ciliary muscle
myopia, 33, 41, 55, 90; *34*

near vision, 20–1, 37, 83
night blindness, 106

oculists, 18
ointment, 30–1
operations, 29; cataract, 76–8; corneal
graft, 49; glaucoma, 69–70, 71;
retinal detachment, 91; squints, 62
ophthalmologists, 18
optic nerves, 9, 12, 63–4, 105, 107
opticians, 18
orthoptists, 18
'ox eye', 72

pain, 16
patches, squints, 61
patchy loss of vision, 13, 14–15
peripheral vision, 14, 21, 106
photochromic lenses, 41, 75
pilocarpine, 66–7, 68
pinguecula, 48
polaroid lenses, 40
presbyopia, 35, 43; *35*
pterygium, 48
ptosis, 17
pupil, 10

radiation injuries, 92
reading: for the blind, 112–13; failing
sight, 108–9; glasses, 35, 36, 41;
lighting, 75–6, 108; *76, 77*
recurrent erosion, 88–9
red eyes, 44–8, 56, 72
refraction, 36–7
registration, blind and partially sighted,
110
retina, 9, 10–12; detachment, 14, 15,
19, 87, 90–1; and diabetes, 97–8;
glaucoma, 63; light sensitivity, 102;
loss of vision, 13–14, 15; macular
degeneration, 82–4; retinitis
pigmentosa, 106–7, 109
rheumatoid arthritis, 44, 50
rods, 10–12

sarcoidosis, 50
sclera, 10
shingles, 16, 50
short sight, 33, 41, 55, 90; *34*
side vision, 14, 21, 106
spectacles, *see* glasses
spots in vision, 99
spring catarrh, 47
squints, 17, 29, 56, 58–62, 105; *57, 60*
steam bathing, 52; *53*
strokes, 15, 17, 21, 103–4; *104*
styes, 17, 23, 51, 56; *52*